Preventing Hospital Infections

Preventing Hospital Infections

Real-World Problems,
Realistic Solutions

SANJAY SAINT
SARAH L. KREIN
WITH
ROBERT W. STOCK

OXFORD
UNIVERSITY PRESS

Oxford University Press is a department of the University of
Oxford. It furthers the University's objective of excellence in research,
scholarship, and education by publishing worldwide.

Oxford   New York

Auckland   Cape Town   Dar es Salaam   Hong Kong   Karachi
Kuala Lumpur   Madrid   Melbourne   Mexico City   Nairobi
New Delhi   Shanghai   Taipei   Toronto

With offices in

Argentina   Austria   Brazil   Chile   Czech Republic   France   Greece
Guatemala   Hungary   Italy   Japan   Poland   Portugal   Singapore
South Korea   Switzerland   Thailand   Turkey   Ukraine   Vietnam

Oxford is a registered trademark of Oxford University Press
in the UK and certain other countries.

Published in the United States of America by
Oxford University Press
198 Madison Avenue, New York, NY 10016

Library of Congress Cataloging-in-Publication Data

Saint, Sanjay, author.
Preventing hospital infections : real-world problems, realistic solutions / Sanjay Saint, Sarah L. Krein ; with Robert W. Stock.
p. ; cm.
Includes bibliographical references.
ISBN 978-0-19-939883-6 (alk. paper)
I. Krein, Sarah L., author.   II. Stock, Robert W., author.   III. Title.
[DNLM: 1. Cross Infection—prevention & control.   2. Catheter-Related Infections—prevention &
control.   3. Equipment Contamination—prevention & control.   4. Guideline Adherence. 5. Infection Control
Practitioners.   6. Infectious Disease Transmission, Professional-to-Patient—prevention & control. WX 167]
RC111
616.9—dc23
2014019487

9 8 7 6 5 4 3
Printed in the United States of America
on acid-free paper

To Veronica, Sean, Kirin, Shaila, Mona, Prem, & Raksha Saint
Sanjay Saint

To my family and to America's Veterans
Sarah L. Krein

To Caryl
Robert W. Stock

CONTENTS

PREFACE   ix

ABOUT THE AUTHORS   xiii

1. A New Strategy to Combat Hospital Infections   1

2. Committing to an Infection Prevention Initiative   9

3. Types of Interventions   20

4. Building the Team   37

5. The Importance of Leadership and Followership   53

6. Common Problems, Realistic Solutions   70

7. Toward Sustainability   91

8. The Collaborative Approach to Preventing Infection   100

9. Taking on *C. Difficile*   111

10. The Future of Infection Prevention   124

REFERENCES   141

INDEX   149

Nearly 2 million Americans develop a healthcare-associated infection each year, and some 100,000 of them die as a result. Yet healthcare-associated infections are reasonably preventable through hospitals' adoption and implementation of evidence-based methods that offer sizable potential savings—in terms of both lives and dollars. A major stumbling block exists between these preventive methods and their full implementation, namely, the failure of large numbers of healthcare personnel to put the methods into practice.

There is no shortage of books that address healthcare-associated infection and its prevention. Most of them, however, are primarily focused on identifying and describing the various types of infection and on the technical aspects of prevention—the sanitary conditions or the latest device that will stop germs from spreading. The adaptive aspects, the acceptance and use of preventive measures by clinical personnel, receive relatively little attention.

This book, to the best of our knowledge, is the first to be primarily devoted to that issue, providing detailed guidance for dealing with the human equation in a hospital quality improvement initiative. We address that challenge in every element of an initiative, from the decision by leadership to proceed, to the selection of a project manager and physician and nurse champions, to the piloting of the initiative on a single medical unit and its roll out to the entire hospital, to the agenda for sustaining the project's gains. There are chapters that pinpoint the main categories of resistance to an initiative and how to cope with them, that analyze the role of leadership in a change initiative, and that explore the future of infection prevention.

In form, the book follows an infection prevention initiative as it might unfold in a model hospital. Because the initiative example addresses catheter-associated urinary tract infection (CAUTI), it involves the entire hospital and the whole range of clinical staff, rather than being limited to, say, the emergency department or intensive care unit. As a result, we believe its lessons can be applied to many other kinds of quality improvement efforts such as those to prevent venous thromboembolism, pressure ulcers, and falls.

The book is relatively concise and written in a conversational style. Its content largely reflects our findings and the work that we have been engaged in over the last decade in trying to understand why some hospitals are more successful than others in preventing healthcare-associated infection. This includes research and prevention-related activities funded by the Department of Veterans Affairs (VA), the National Institutes of Health (NIH), the Agency for Healthcare Research and Quality (AHRQ), the Blue Cross Blue Shield of Michigan Foundation, and the Michigan Health and Hospital Association Keystone Center.

In addition to the valuable support of our funders, we have been fortunate to work with a terrific group of individuals who share our goal of preventing infection and enhancing patient safety. We are ever grateful to our dedicated project staff including Elissa Gaies, Karen Fowler, Molly Harrod, Hiroko Kiyoshi-Teo, Edward Kennedy, Debbie Zawol, Karen Belanger, Jane Forman, Christine Kowalski, Todd Greene, Laura Damschroder, Latoya Kuhn, Andy Hickner, David Ratz, John Colozzi, Heidi Reichert, and Brenda Hoelzer. We have benefited greatly from our fruitful collaborations with a large number of individuals from different parts of the world including Tim Hofer, Jennifer Meddings, Jane Banaszak-Holl, Mohamad Fakih, Russ Olmsted, Anne Sales, Mary Rogers, Emily Shuman, Milisa Manojlovich, Lona Mody, Sam Watson, Barbara Trautner, Joel Howell, Scott Flanders, Vineet Chopra, Hugo Sax, Benedetta Allegranzi, Alessandro Bartoloni, Akihiko Saitoh, Didier Pittet, John Hollingsworth, Carol Chenoweth, Nathorn Chaiyakunapruk, Laraine Washer, Carolyn Gould, Anucha Apisarnthanarak, Ben Lipsky, Bob Wachter, Ken Langa, Matt Samore, Jim Battles, Steve Hines, Barbara Edson, and Yasuharu Tokuda.

We also appreciate the support we have received from our employers: the VA Ann Arbor Healthcare System and the University of Michigan. Both are organizations that are committed to excellence in all that they do and we are honored to call both organizations our home. We remain grateful to our many supervisors through the years who have provided us with the support and encouragement to conduct our work including Rod Hayward, Larry McMahon, John Carethers, Rich Moseley, Eve Kerr, John Del Valle, Eric Young, Mike Finegan, and Robert McDivitt. We also thank the many healthcare providers and administrators who participated in our interviews and shared with us their stories (trials, tribulations, and successes) as they worked to prevent infections in their hospitals. It is these individuals and their counterparts in hospitals across the United States and the world for whom this book is primarily intended as we collectively strive to improve the safety of hospitalized patients.

So, let the journey begin!

Sanjay Saint
Sarah L. Krein
Robert W. Stock

ABOUT THE AUTHORS

Sanjay Saint, MD, MPH, is the George Dock Professor of Internal Medicine at the University of Michigan, the Director of the VA/University of Michigan Patient Safety Enhancement Program, and the Associate Chief of Medicine at the VA Ann Arbor Healthcare System. His research focuses on enhancing patient safety by preventing healthcare-associated infection and translating research findings into practice. He has authored over 250 peer-reviewed papers with approximately 80 appearing in the *New England Journal of Medicine, JAMA, Lancet,* or the *Annals of Internal Medicine.* He is an international leader in preventing catheter-associated urinary tract infection (CAUTI) and is currently on the leadership team of a federally funded project that aims to reduce CAUTI across the United States. He is a special correspondent to the *New England Journal of Medicine,* an editorial board member of the *Annals of Internal Medicine,* and an elected member of the American Society for Clinical Investigation. He received his Medical Doctorate from the University of California at Los Angeles, completed a medical residency and chief residency at the University of California at San Francisco, and obtained a Masters in Public Health (as a Robert Wood Johnson Clinical Scholar) from the University of Washington in Seattle. He has been a visiting professor at over 50 universities and hospitals in the United States, Europe, and Japan, and has active research studies underway with investigators in Switzerland, Italy, Japan, Australia, and Thailand.

Sarah L. Krein, PhD, RN, is a Research Associate Professor of Internal Medicine at the University of Michigan and a Research Health Science Specialist at the VA Ann Arbor Center for Clinical Management Research (a VA HSR&D Center of Innovation). She also has an adjunct appointment at the University of Michigan School of Nursing. Dr. Krein received her BSN from the University of Mary in Bismarck, ND, and her PhD in Health

Services Research from the University of Minnesota in Minneapolis, MN. Dr. Krein's research interests include organizational behavior and implementation research with a particular focus on enhancing patient safety and preventing healthcare-associated complications. Her research is funded through grants and contracts from the Department of Veterans Affairs, the National Institutes of Health, and the Agency for Healthcare Research and Quality.

Robert W. Stock is a freelance book and magazine writer. As an editor, writer, and columnist for The *New York Times* for three decades, and as a freelancer, he has frequently written about medical subjects, ranging from amniocentesis to genetic counseling to public health.

Preventing Hospital Infections

A New Strategy to Combat Hospital Infections

The hospital is altogether the most complex human organization ever devised.

—Peter Drucker

W e were interviewing staff members at a dozen hospitals that had taken part in a campaign to reduce healthcare-associated urinary tract infections. The goal was to make sure that indwelling urinary catheters were only used when medically necessary and were removed promptly when no longer needed. Sounds simple enough, but it turned out to be infinitely complex, and confusing.

We discovered, for example, that there were two sets of nurses who were worried about their patients taking a fall. One set wanted the catheter out as soon as possible because it interfered with patient mobility and they feared that their patients, especially those who are a bit confused and do not even realize the catheter is in place, might trip on the tubing. "They are going to try and get out of bed and injure themselves," one nurse said.

Another set of nurses favored maintaining the catheter in place as long as possible because it tended to keep their patients in bed. A nurse, quoted by an infection preventionist, put it this way: "Well, do I really want this person hopping out of bed and can I really be sure that they're going to call me to help them? We don't want there to be any falls."

Two groups of nurses, both concerned about their patients' well-being, but one group gladly cooperated with an infection prevention program, while the other group was, at best, reluctant. As is so often true when a hospital embarks on a campaign to control infection, the human dimension intruded.

There is universal agreement within the nation's hospitals that the prevention of healthcare-associated infection (HAI) is an absolute necessity for both humane and financial reasons. And there is no shortage of evidence-based strategies that can take us closer to that goal. Studies[1,2] have demonstrated that at least 20% of all healthcare-associated infections can be prevented, and some researchers have suggested that the figure might reach 70%. Yet many of the efforts that hospitals have made to implement these proven strategies have fallen short of their goals. Why? Our research has shown that a principal reason is the failure of the hospitals to win their staffs' active support of the infection prevention initiatives. In their focus on the technical aspects of an initiative, these hospitals have given short shrift to the human aspects.

This book offers a field-tested framework for organizing and implementing a hospital-based initiative to combat infection. It includes descriptions and explanations of some evidence-based infection prevention procedures, but the major focus is on ways to inspire full-scale adoption of these practices: essentially, to change behavior. We answer this central question: Given all the complexities of the hospital operation—the hierarchical arrangements, the competing priorities, the web of personal relationships—how do you get the people of a hospital to truly buy into an infection prevention initiative?

The stakes are high, and they can be quickly stated. The Centers for Disease Control and Prevention (CDC) estimate that there were 722,000 hospital-acquired infections in 2011, leading to 75,000 fatalities.[3] The annual direct medical cost of healthcare-associated infections to hospitals is an estimated $40 billion.[4] The infections create physical and emotional distress for hundreds of thousands of patients annually. They also take a psychological toll on the staff of a hospital and on its culture, constant reminders of their failure to live up to their credo, *primum non nocere*—first, do no harm.

Hospitals have not been ignoring the problem, far from it. Spurred on by a consumer-driven patient safety movement, they have undertaken hundreds of programs to combat HAI, providing a classic example of the translation of medical research findings into clinical practice and better care for the patient. And the programs have had an impact: The CDC infection and fatality figures previously cited are considerably lower than earlier estimates.

At one hospital, the scene of a campaign to reduce infections caused by central venous catheters, we interviewed an infection preventionist who wanted to extend the campaign from the intensive care unit (ICU) to the operating room. At a management Christmas party, over cocktails, he asked the head of anesthesiology whether he was aware that, with the ICU project in full swing, the operating room was now the source of all of the hospital's central venous catheter infections. The anesthesiologist was surprised and chagrined and, in short order, a convert to extending the campaign to his bailiwick.

"My philosophy," the preventionist said, "has always been: What if it's your mother, your father? We always want the best care for those that we love and we try to bring that home to everyone in the hospital."

But our hospitals as a whole have a long way to go before they realize their infection prevention goals. A recent national study of the status of infection prevention in approximately 1,500 U.S. ICUs made that all too evident.[5] Overall, reported staff adherence to prevention practices for the three most common device-related infections—central line-associated bloodstream infection (CLABSI), ventilator-associated pneumonia (VAP), and catheter-associated urinary tract infection (CAUTI)—was quite variable and, in some cases, depressingly low. For CLABSI, reported adherence to prevention policies ranged from 37% to 71%, adherence to VAP prevention policies ranged from 45% to 55%, and adherence to CAUTI prevention policies was between 6% and 27%.

In addition, there have been government initiatives on state and federal levels. In 2009, for example, the Department of Health and Human Services launched a nationwide action plan, increasing its financial support of HAI-related projects and setting five-year goals for a major reduction of five of the most serious hospital-acquired infections. The Centers for Medicare and Medicaid Services (CMS) has stopped reimbursing hospitals for the extra costs involved in treating a number of hospital infections. Starting in 2014, all CMS payments to hospitals "that rank in the lowest-performing quartile of hospital-acquired conditions," including some infections, have been reduced by 1%. And CMS requires that hospitals report their infection rates for several HAIs, information that is critical to understanding how best to target such infections.

The two healthcare-affiliated authors of this book have, individually and jointly, closely observed, participated in, and published academic papers about a number of effective efforts to combat hospital infections. Sanjay Saint, MD, MPH, is the George Dock Professor of Medicine at the University of Michigan, Ann Arbor, and Associate Chief of Medicine at the VA Ann Arbor Healthcare System. Sarah Krein, PhD, RN, is a Research Associate Professor of Internal Medicine as well as an Adjunct Research Associate Professor at the University's School of Nursing and a Research Investigator at the VA Ann Arbor Healthcare System.

Though they inhabit the same healthcare universe, nurses and doctors often have very different perspectives as to how that universe should and should not operate. As the economist and healthcare writer Gerhard Kocher put it, "Nursing would be a dream job if there were no doctors." Nevertheless, the authors have amicably managed to combine their varying perspectives in their research and in the creation of this book.

Both of them, for example, were part of the leadership group in a statewide initiative sponsored by the Michigan Health and Hospital Association to reduce CAUTI. Between January 2007 and March 2012, the campaign achieved a 30% decrease in the number of patients with urinary catheters, a reduction of 25% in urinary tract infections, and savings of $10 million.[6]

Healthcare-associated infections caused by such indwelling devices are especially common—and preventable. They have thus become the leading edge of efforts to combat HAI. In this book, we will be using the following three devices to illustrate our themes:

- Ventilator, also known as a respirator. Pneumonia strikes 10% to 20% of patients on a ventilator for more than two days and doubles their risk of dying.
- Central venous catheter, also known as a central line. Infections from the use of these catheters, which remain in place near the heart for several weeks or more, are also life-threatening. They affect up to 120,000 hospitalized patients a year.[3]
- Indwelling urinary catheter, also known as a Foley. Infections associated with this catheter, though generally less dangerous than the other two conditions, create serious pain and discomfort for patients, and account for the majority of the roughly 175,000 annual urinary tract infections—making it the most common device-associated infection in the United States.[3]

In all three cases, "bundles" of clinical interventions for preventing infection have been developed. Though these interventions vary in their details, they share the common goal of removing the device as soon as possible.

* * *

The infection prevention framework we present in the chapters to come is focused on CAUTI, rather than VAP or CLABSI. Hospitals have found CAUTI far more resistant to quality improvement efforts than the other two infections. We also believe that the CAUTI prevention framework can serve a larger purpose, as a model for coping with a variety of other hospital challenges, including the prevention of falls, pressure ulcers, and *Clostridium difficile* infection.

In the quotation that opens this chapter, Peter Drucker marvels at the complexity of the hospital as an organization. The CAUTI model can help us unravel some of that complexity and gain a better understanding of hospitals' operations.

Why is a CAUTI prevention framework an apt model for this larger role? Several reasons:

- CAUTI's impact on patients is felt throughout the hospital, from the emergency department to the medical-surgical floor to the rehab unit to the ICU—unlike VAP and CLABSI, for instance, which are found primarily among the critically ill.
- CAUTI prevention involves a broad spectrum of hospital personnel, including nurses, physicians, infection preventionists, administrators, nursing aides, and microbiologists.
- CAUTI can easily fly under the radar in an environment governed by the rule of rescue, where heart attacks and other life-threatening events trump all else. The same is true of several other hospital-acquired conditions.
- The CAUTI model relies heavily on widely applicable socio-adaptive concerns, rather than on technical elements that vary with each target problem. For example, frontline clinicians must be truly engaged and positive communication fostered between nurses and physicians, essential goals shared by so many other quality improvement efforts.

The basic framework of the CAUTI model can be used to combat a variety of infections, including those caused by the more than 30 species of the *Staphylococcus*, commonly referred to as "*Staph*," bacteria. *Staph* infections range from the mild, such as a simple boil, to the potentially fatal, such as methicillin-resistant *Staphylococcus aureus* (MRSA). The framework is also an appropriate model for preventing "sepsis," which can occur because of the immune system's destructive reaction to an infection. To put it another way, a case of sepsis can happen because a successful infection prevention program did not.

We have chosen the stand-alone hospital as the venue for our discussion of the CAUTI framework rather than a group of hospitals operating as a collaborative. We believe that an infection prevention campaign can be more clearly presented in that context, but we do discuss the collaborative option in detail in Chapter 8.

In the course of our research, we have identified dozens of best practices—reasons why some hospitals have been more successful in preventing infection than others. The strategies and observations, including many of the actual quotes, were drawn from hundreds of interviews of hospital personnel at all levels, conducted through telephone conversations and during site visits to hospitals from Maine to California. Each stage of an infection prevention project is described and analyzed, from the hospital's decision to undertake the campaign to the putting together of a team to lead it to the actual implementation of the campaign on the hospital floor. The barriers to success are many, from nurses who actively resist any change in their routine, to physicians who oppose any kind of new oversight, to administrators who find ways of delaying the delivery of key resources. We suggest concrete techniques to inform the reader's step-by-step, chapter-by-chapter progress toward the goal of a successful—and sustainable—intervention. We also dedicate chapter 9 to describing how the CAUTI prevention framework might be applied to another, quite different challenge: *C. difficile* infection.

The ultimate aspiration for any hospital, of course, is a culture of clinical excellence. We talked about that with the medical director of a highly rated hospital, who explained his approach to quality initiatives: "We just say it's evidence-based. You cannot refute evidence-based medicine, and that's the way we're going to do things." The initiative might take a while because "You're changing habits," he said, "but we just keep beating on it."

SUGGESTIONS FOR FURTHER READING

Cardo, D., Dennehy, P. H., Halverson, P., Fishman, N., Kohn, M., Murphy, C. L., . . . HAI Elimination White Paper Writing Group. (2010). Moving toward elimination of healthcare-associated infections: A call to action. *American Journal of Infection Control, 38*(9), 671–675.

In this 2010 collaborative call to action, multiple professional societies and governmental agencies, including the Centers for Disease Control and Prevention, lay out a plan for the elimination of healthcare-associated infection. This article presents the following general issues that continue to be at the center of prevention-related efforts: (a) adherence to evidence-based practices; (b) alignment of incentives; (c) innovation through basic, translational, and epidemiological research; and (d) data to target prevention efforts and measure progress.

Pronovost, P., Needham, D., Berenholtz, S., Sinopoli, D., Chu, H., Cosgrove, S., . . . Goeschel, C. (2006). An intervention to decrease catheter-related bloodstream infections in the ICU. *New England Journal of Medicine, 355*(26), 2725–2732.

In this cohort study of 103 ICUs in Michigan, Pronovost and colleagues found that an evidence-based intervention resulted in a decreased rate of catheter-related bloodstream infection per 1,000 catheter-days from 2.7 infections at baseline to 0 infections at 3 months post-implementation, and that the mean rate per 1,000 catheter-days decreased from 7.7 at baseline to 1.4 at 16 to 18 months of follow-up.

Saint, S., Howell, J. D., & Krein, S.L. (2010). Implementation science: How to jump start infection prevention. *Infection Control and Hospital Epidemiology, 31*(Suppl. 1), S14–S17.

By suggesting a conceptual framework and other key strategies for translating infection prevention evidence into practice, the authors explore infection prevention as a paradigm for implementation science.

Saint, S., Meddings, J. A., Calfee, D. P., Kowalski, C. P., & Krein, S. L. (2009). Catheter-associated urinary tract infection and the Medicare rule changes. *Annals of Internal Medicine, 150,* 877–885.

This article explores the 2008 changes in reimbursement by the Centers for Medicare & Medicaid Services as they apply to catheter-associated urinary tract infection (CAUTI). The authors provide an overview of CAUTI prevention and the rule changes, as well as suggesting consequences, practical implications, and next steps for hospitals.

Saint, S., Olmsted, R. N., Fakih, M. G., Kowalski, C. P., Watson, S. R., Sales, A. E., & Krein, S. L. (2009). Translating health care-associated urinary tract infection research into practice via the bladder bundle. *Joint Commission Journal on Quality and Patient Safety, 35*(9), 449–455.

In this article, the authors present an overview of the "bladder bundle initiative" in Michigan. The initiative focused on preventing catheter-associated urinary tract infection by optimizing the use of urinary catheters with a specific emphasis on continual assessment and catheter removal as soon as possible, especially for patients without a clear indication. Their observations suggest that simply disseminating scientific evidence is often ineffective in changing clinical practice and, therefore, that learning how to implement these findings is critically important to promoting high-quality care and a safe healthcare environment.

Committing to an Infection Prevention Initiative

I think one's feelings waste themselves in words; they ought all to be distilled into actions which bring results.

—FLORENCE NIGHTINGALE

"Everyone is interested in quality," the hospital epidemiologist said, explaining why her hospital's leaders had supported an initiative to combat infection, "but the reason behind the interest in quality is not because we're incredibly nice people. It's because if you don't save money, you're going to be bankrupt."

Of course, it's never quite that simple. Like every organization run by human beings, hospitals make decisions in response to a wide variety of carrots and sticks. Financial incentives are an important factor, but far from the only ones. And what makes the equation even more complex is how individual hospitals differ from each other because of such factors as their size, the nature of their patient population, and (there it is again) their financial circumstances.

Along with those factors, though, and influenced by them, is a hospital's level of commitment to excellence in patient care. Over the last few decades, to an important degree, that level of commitment has come to be defined by a hospital's willingness to undertake infection prevention initiatives. Such interventions have saved thousands of patients' lives and saved millions more from various kinds of misery. But the infection threat has grown worse.

Multi-drug resistant organisms (MDROs) are proliferating around the globe. Infection prevention efforts in hospitals—such as those reducing the use of indwelling catheters—keep deadly MDROs like methicillin-resistant *Staphylococcus aureus* (MRSA) out of the bloodstream, and they eliminate the need to use and overuse antimicrobials. Thus, hospital leaders may also approve infection prevention interventions because of the threat that infection poses to their patients; the C-suite actually does house a number of "incredibly nice people."

WHY HOSPITALS SIGN ON

In this chapter, we explore the reasons that hospital officials take on infection prevention initiatives, and how they get the ball rolling.

Sometimes the infection prevention decision is part of a package, a larger systems redesign. Many hospitals have adopted a Lean or a Six Sigma approach aimed at improving overall operational efficiency. Hospital CEOs recognize that forestalling infection is eminently efficient, as well as humane.

In other cases, CEOs call for an infection prevention intervention because they learn that their hospitals' infection rate has been rising above the national norm—or above the rate achieved by nearby competitors. Hospitals in the same area compete for customers—or "patients," as we call them—at least as energetically as any neighborhood stores. They can't afford to fall behind. And now that hospitals' infection rates, along with other measures, have become a matter of public knowledge—via the Centers for Medicare & Medicaid Services' (CMS) Hospital Compare website, for example, and some state websites—administrators have a powerful new motivation for keeping up with the Joneses. In December 2013, the website added MRSA and *C. difficile* to its list of publicly reported healthcare-associated infections (HAIs). (A claim to being a town's "safest hospital" can be a powerful marketing tool.)

By the same token, many a CEO has got religion about infection prevention when the hospital down the street announced plans for a major quality initiative or agreed to join in a statewide collaborative project to lower infection rates. As we will discuss in Chapter 8, collaboratives can exert a powerful magnetic force on a hospital, even though they typically force the staff to jump through any number of hoops.

The impetus for an intervention may also come from within the institution. An intensivist returns from an Institute for Healthcare Improvement conference touting the benefits of a new twist on ventilator-associated pneumonia (VAP) prevention or the critical care oversight committee develops a proposal for an intervention to reduce the incidence of catheter-associated urinary tract infection (CAUTI). Sometimes the genesis of an initiative arises from the ranks of hospital employees, from someone like a nurse we interviewed, a specialist in placing the peripherally inserted central catheter (PICC).

She described her reaction after learning of her hospital's sky-high central line-associated bloodstream infection (CLABSI) rate. "I was literally crying, tearing my hair out," she said. She asked herself, "What can I do?"

She began by convincing her supervisor to give her an assistant so she would have time to teach nurses at the bedside how to better care for the central lines. She lobbied for time off to research CLABSI prevention, and began introducing evidence-based measures to combat the infection. After her campaign was brought to the attention of the hospital's leadership, her prevention approach was adopted in all the hospital's intensive care units (ICUs), and central line infection rates plummeted from 4 per 1,000 catheter days to 1.2.

More typically, an infection prevention intervention starts with the infection prevention staff. They are the people, after all, who collect, analyze, and interpret a hospital's infection data and report the results to hospital personnel and local, state, and federal authorities. They are the first to see negative trends developing in a hospital and among the first to learn about new scientific prevention developments.

Hospital leaders lean toward infection prevention initiatives when the moves are backed by science. An infection preventionist, describing how he presents a proposal for an initiative to management, told us, "We really work at providing evidence-based practices as opposed to, 'This is the new gadget out there; we should go with it.'" And the leadership responds to appeals to patient safety. But one of the biggest sticks among the carrots and sticks that influence CEOs is wielded by the federal government and it carries a dollar sign.

CMS INCENTIVES

The CMS decision to stop reimbursing hospitals for the extra cost of healthcare-associated infections, joined in by commercial insurers, has given the C-suite a powerful extra incentive to fight those infections. One hospital study[1] found that, prior to the October 2008 enforcement of that decision, a Medicare inpatient with pneumonia would have yielded a CMS payment of $6,072 if there were no complications; $8,346 if there was also a CAUTI, and $11,891 if there was a renal abscess associated with a urinary catheter. Now, CMS pays just the initial $6,072 (in 2008 dollars), and the hospital must absorb the difference. (See Box 2.1.)

A survey of infection preventionists, published in 2012,[2] found that 81% of respondents had observed a greater focus since 2008 on the infections targeted by CMS, and nearly 70% were spending more time educating

---

Box 2.1

To estimate the current cost of CAUTI to their individual institutions, hospitals can access a "CAUTI Cost Calculator" on www.catheterout. org, a website developed by the authors and associates at the VA Ann Arbor Healthcare System and the University of Michigan. The calculator can also be used to estimate the projected costs following a hypothetical intervention to reduce Foley use.

staff on best practices to prevent CLABSI and CAUTI. The survey also discovered that about 50% of respondents said they were spending more time working with physicians and coders to document infections that were present upon a patient's *admission* to the hospital. No point in getting stung for infections that occurred before the patient even arrived!

There are, in fact, some serious concerns about how CMS decides these reimbursements, especially its use of "claims" (sometimes referred to as "administrative") data generated from physicians' notes. Those notes rarely contain the text that coders require to label a urinary tract infection as catheter-associated or hospital-acquired in billing data. So the rate of CAUTI claims is much lower than epidemiological studies and surveillance data suggest it should be. We believe that claims data are not valid for imposing the CMS penalties on HAI, nor are they valid for comparing hospitals in public reporting for healthcare-associated complication rates. Hospitals with higher complication rates in claims data may simply be better at documenting those conditions, or have a patient population more susceptible to infection. Fortunately, a recent decision from the federal government addresses these issues. Beginning October 1, 2014, quality measures and scoring methodology have been improved, specifically for CLABSI and CAUTI rates. Rather than base rates on claims data, the CMS will look to the National Healthcare Safety Network (NHSN) database to determine reimbursement levels. Also, the CMS system now takes into account a patient's age, gender, and comorbid conditions so that hospitals that cater to sicker patients are not penalized. These modifications represent changes in the correct direction.

CMS has also provided hospital administrators with other financial incentives to undertake quality improvement initiatives. Hospitals that perform in the bottom 25% in their prevention of several patient complications are subject to a penalty on their overall Medicare payments—1% as of fiscal year 2015 (which begins on October 1, 2014). The complications range from some HAIs and late-stage pressure ulcers to foreign objects left in patients after surgery. And CMS rewards hospitals that are in the top quartile in their prevention of complications—increasing payments by 1% as of fiscal year 2015.

Though financial matters loom large when a hospital determines whether to initiate an infection prevention program, they should not be the ultimate influence. That role belongs to the essential culture of the institution. Is the hospital fully committed to quality patient care as its core mission? Does that concern for the patient weigh heavily in the leaders' major decisions?

In the course of our research, we found a large public hospital that came close to meeting those standards. The fact that the staff served a largely poverty-stricken patient population actually seemed to nurture a patient-centered approach.

"There's a bunch of homeless folks that come here," the chief of staff told us, "so it's a real 'get-down-and-get-dirty' kind of place. But everybody loves to be here, whether you're in OB or you're psych or you're peds, because they get a chance to make a difference in peoples' lives . . . "

A quality manager at this hospital added that the staff had to be "as nice as we can be to some people who aren't very nice to us, so it just takes a special kind of person to be down here, and I think that's why it works."

The chief executive officer, staff members told us, was another essential element in the hospital's success, in part because she is a nurse with a deep understanding of what happens on the patient floors, and in part because of her patient-centered, collaborative management style. Several people described the culture of the hospital as "collegial" and "egalitarian." Nurses serve on all of the medical staff committees, and all the other committees have doctor members. The chief of staff described the workings of the critical care committee, which he said includes doctors, nurses, and "everybody else." For things to happen, he went on, requires agreement across the board: "It's like an end-of-life discussion where the decision is made with everybody on the same page."

This is the same institution that was mobilized by the PICC nurse to undertake the program to prevent CLABSI. What counted was not the source of the idea but its validity as a means of improving patient care.

When we asked that hospital's epidemiologist about his institution's culture, he replied, "Striving for excellence would be a fair way to describe it." That's also a fair description of the model hospital that will be making a regular appearance in the chapters to come. This midsize, 250-bed facility, an entity entirely of our own invention, is intended to serve as a framework on which to hang dozens of infection prevention best practices.

To be sure, for any given challenge, there are all sorts of potential solutions that may be better or worse, depending on the particular circumstances and the nature of the particular hospital and its staff. We will be presenting a host of such solutions along the way, but we also wanted to provide a coherent, step-by-step picture of how a successful infection prevention initiative might be conducted—starting with the decision to proceed.

THE CEO MAKES A DECISION

At the model hospital, that decision has been generated at the top. The chief executive officer, cognizant of the CMS pressure on the financial side and the need to reduce infections, consults with his clinical leaders. They agree to take on a small package of initiatives covering CAUTI, VAP, and CLABSI prevention.

Next question: Who, from among the leadership, is going to oversee each initiative? The project sponsor has to be willing and able to take on this extra responsibility. It is not likely to consume all that much of his or her time, but there will be some initial meetings and a steady stream of reports to look over. A project manager will have to be found to be the operational leader. And the sponsor will be called on if and when the initiative triggers disputes or problems that cannot be resolved in the lower ranks.

At the model hospital, the chief executive officer and the chief of staff (otherwise known as the chief medical officer or vice president of medical affairs) call in the director of critical care for a heart-to-heart. They urge him to accept executive sponsorship of the VAP and CLABSI initiatives, which will be focused in the hospital's two intensive care units, one medical and the other surgical. The director points out that the interventions will require some major changes in practice that could strain his department's budget, but in the end he agrees to take on the extra job. In any event, he expects the nurses and physicians in charge of each ICU to run their own programs.

The chief executive officer turns the CAUTI initiative over to the chief nursing executive since the focus of this initiative will involve changing the hospital's bedside nursing practice. With her top deputy, the director of nursing, the chief nursing executive goes over a list of potential sponsors, including the head of quality and the chief infection preventionist. The head of quality, they decide, is too academic, too removed from the problems of the wards. The infection preventionist, though she has a solid reputation among both physicians and nurses, has no experience in bedside nursing care. They know that in order to get buy-in from the floor nurses, it will be imperative to have someone who has "walked the talk." The chief nurse finally urges her deputy, the director of nursing, to become the project's executive sponsor—and receives the answer she hoped for.

In her role as executive sponsor, the director of nursing understands that even though the CAUTI initiative has the support of the hospital's leaders, they have many other concerns—projects and challenges that may have a higher priority. She knows that she will probably have to battle to obtain extra funding for some aspects of the intervention, primarily new products like portable ultrasounds and perhaps even overtime as nurses struggle to learn a new way of dealing with indwelling catheters. They will be following a checklist of behaviors embodied in the bladder bundle, an evidence-based collection of do's and don'ts. (See Box 2.2.)

If the model hospital runs true to form, the executive sponsor realizes there will be plenty of staff opposition to the intervention. The history of quality improvement is filled with tales of people, set in their ways, who ridiculed such changes as the presurgery time-out until it saved them from embarrassing error. Now a standard of care, the time-out requires the verbal identification of every aspect of the procedure from the names of the patient and participants to the name of the procedure and its location on the patient.

More recently, many hospitals have encountered a refusal by a substantial percentage of their staff to obey hand hygiene rules, despite their

---

Box 2.2 RECOMMENDATIONS FOR PREVENTING CATHETER-ASSOCIATED URINARY TRACT INFECTION: "ABCDE" (ADAPTED FROM SAINT ET AL.[3])

- **A**septic catheter insertion and proper maintenance is paramount.
- **B**ladder ultrasound may avoid indwelling catheterization.
- **C**ondom catheters or other alternatives to an indwelling catheter such as intermittent catheterization should be considered in appropriate patients.
- **D**o not use the indwelling catheter unless you must!
- **E**arly removal of the catheter using a reminder or nurse-initiated removal protocol when it appears warranted.

---

proven efficacy. Some hospitals have installed elaborate technological aids to check up on staff adherence to the rules. In one example, a video camera records whether people entering an intensive care room wash their hands. In another example, staffers wear badges that vibrate when they approach a patient's bed if they have failed to wash their hands. To outwit the devices, some hidebound staffers have ducked under waist-high monitors and turned on the water in the room's sink to avoid a badge reaction but without washing their hands.[4]

At the model hospital, the executive sponsor is happily aware that she will not personally have to impose a new Foley procedure on the staff. That will be the task of the project manager and his or her team, including a nurse champion and a physician champion. The sponsor will have to find a project manager, who will, in turn, assemble the team.

The sponsor actually has a candidate in mind, one of her own—a veteran unit manager who has put together a model inpatient nursing unit. She is assertive when necessary and she knows what buttons to push. She also has a full measure of the needed interpersonal skills: she is patient, persistent, and enthusiastic about improving patient care, and she has built positive relationships with many of the hospital's nurses and physicians in the course of managing previous quality initiatives. Before the sponsor talks with her, though, she consults with the chief nursing executive, winning her approval.

In the chapters ahead, our description of the model hospital will mainly focus on its CAUTI prevention effort as a best-practice example, although we will also discuss the particular personnel challenges of the VAP and CLABSI initiatives. Our goal throughout is to offer field-tested insights to aid in the adoption and implementation of quality improvement initiatives.

SUGGESTIONS FOR FURTHER READING

Burke, J. P. (2003). Infection control—a problem for patient safety. *New England Journal of Medicine, 348*(7), 651–656.

> In this article, Burke discusses the major problems in infection control, approaches for solving these problems, the role of the National Nosocomial Infections Surveillance System of the Centers for Disease Control and Prevention (precursor to the current National Healthcare Safety Network System) as a model, and the need for renewed commitment to, and innovations in, infection control to help ensure patient safety. This was one of the first articles that linked infection prevention and control to patient safety.

Hollingsworth, J. M., Rogers, M. A., Krein, S. L., Hickner, A., Kuhn, L., Cheng, A., . . . Saint, S. (2013). Determining the noninfectious complications of indwelling urethral catheters: A systematic review and meta-analysis. *Annals of Internal Medicine, 159*(6), 401–410.

> In this systematic review and meta-analysis, Hollingsworth and colleagues pooled 37 studies (2,868 patients) to determine the frequency of noninfectious complications after indwelling urinary catheterization. They concluded that many noninfectious catheter-associated complications (urine leakage, urethral strictures, and gross hematuria) were at least as common as clinically significant urinary tract infections. These results suggest that it is important to consider these possible harms as well as CAUTI when targeting prevention efforts.

Saint, S., Kowalski, C. P., Kaufman, S. R., Hofer, T. P., Kauffman, C. A., Olmsted, R. N., & Krein, S. L. (2008). Preventing hospital-acquired urinary tract infection in the United States: A national study. *Clinical Infectious Diseases, 46*(2), 243–250.

> In this national study, the authors surveyed 600 non-VA and 119 VA hospitals to better understand the current practices used to prevent healthcare-associated urinary tract infection (UTI). They found that 56% of hospitals did not have a system for monitoring those patients who had urinary catheters in place and 74% did not monitor catheter duration. Overall, they found no widely used strategy (e.g., bladder scanners, catheter reminders, or condom catheters) to prevent

healthcare-associated UTIs. These results suggest that despite the knowledge that there is a strong link between urinary catheters and subsequent UTIs, there are many evidence-based practices that are not being implemented to prevent catheter-associated complications.

Saint, S., Lipsky, B. A., & Goold, S. D. (2002). Indwelling urinary catheters: A one-point restraint? *Annals of Internal Medicine, 137*(2), 125–127.

In this editorial, the authors discuss the often unjustified and excessively prolonged persistence of urinary catheter use despite clear evidence of its detrimental effects. They discuss the practical effect of needlessly confining patients in what could be called a "one-point" restraint, raising serious safety and ethical concerns analogous to those noted more than a decade ago with "four-point" (limb) restraints and propose that lessons learned from efforts to curtail the use of physical restraints may help identify strategies for diminishing the use of indwelling urinary catheters.

Umscheid, C. A., Mitchell, M. D., Doshi, J. A., Agarwal, R., Williams, K., & Brennan, P. J. (2011). Estimating the proportion of healthcare-associated infections that are reasonably preventable and the related mortality and costs. *Infection Control and Hospital Epidemiology, 32*(2), 101–114.

In this study, Umscheid and colleagues performed a systematic review of interventions to reduce healthcare-associated infections and national data to estimate the preventability of central line-associated bloodstream infection (CLABSI), catheter-associated urinary tract infection (CAUTI), surgical site infection (SSI), and ventilator-associated pneumonia (VAP). They found that as many as 65% to 70% of cases of CLABSI and CAUTI and 55% of cases of VAP and SSI may be preventable with current evidence-based strategies. These results suggest that, although 100% prevention may be unattainable, comprehensive implementation of evidence-based strategies could prevent hundreds of thousands of infections and save tens of thousands of lives and billions of dollars.

Types of Interventions

The great tragedy of science is the slaying of a beautiful hypothesis by an ugly fact.

—Thomas Henry Huxley

Long before there were hospitals, there were healthcare-associated infections, contracted in the course of self-treatment. There has, for example, always been some kind of urinary catheter that a person might use to cope with urinary incontinence and other such difficulties— and some kind of urinary tract infection as a result. In this chapter, our focus is on the basics of infection prevention, current best practices, and such attendant devices as the catheter that represent the technical side of a quality improvement intervention (as opposed to the adaptive, people side). But first, a bit of background, for urinary catheterization has a storied past.

The ancient Chinese relied on onion stalks, whereas the ancient Egyptians and Greeks used tubes of wood and metal, all of them passed through the urethra into the bladder. Benjamin Franklin invented a flexible catheter in 1752 to relieve his brother, John, who had bladder stones, and probably used it somewhat later on himself for the same problem. During the 1930s, Dr. Frederic Eugene Basil Foley was one of several urologists who were developing catheters that had a small, water-inflated balloon on the end that kept the device from slipping out of the body. Eventually, the indwelling balloon catheter was universally adopted, and it was Dr. Foley's name that became permanently attached to the device.

HOSPITALS AND THE GERM THEORY OF DISEASE

For many millions of people, suffering from urinary retention or incontinence or recovering from genitourinary surgery, the catheter can be a godsend. But like any foreign object introduced into the body, be it a central venous catheter or an endotracheal tube attached to a mechanical ventilator, the urinary catheter can introduce dangerous bacteria. The effort to prevent the infections that can arise because of these objects, the subject of this book, is part of a larger, long-running campaign to stave off infection in the hospital setting.

A major milestone in that effort came in the 1840s when a Viennese physician, Ignaz Semmelweis, discovered the cause of a flare-up of puerperal fever in a delivery room. The medical students who were helping with deliveries often arrived in the room directly from performing autopsies—and without properly washing their hands. Once they began washing with a chlorinated lime solution, the death rate in the maternity ward plunged by 500%! When Semmelweis sought to spread word of his discovery, he was ridiculed and forced from his position. In a new post at a different hospital, he confirmed his findings, but the powers-that-be in the healthcare community still rejected his ideas. He eventually became emotionally unstable and died in an insane asylum at the age of 47.

The resistance of the medical profession to change, even such a simple and well-confirmed change, may seem startling in retrospect. And yet, here we are, more than a century-and-a-half later, still struggling to convince hospital personnel to wash their hands regularly. In spite of a full-press international campaign, average hand hygiene rates are only about 40%.[1]

The prevailing wisdom in Semmelweis's time held that disease was spread by foul-smelling and poisonous vapors, miasmas, caused by the rotting of organic substances. Cholera, for example, was thought to be caused by breathing in bad air or drinking contaminated water. Enter Louis Pasteur, the 19th-century French chemist who so famously proved otherwise.

At the time, the process that created wine, beer, and vinegar was thought to be a simple chemical reaction producing yeast as a byproduct. Pasteur showed that, in fact, microorganisms, in this case yeast, were responsible for the fermentation process, and he succeeded in identifying the germs that sometimes fouled up the process—producing sour milk or reducing alcohol production. He further discovered that he could kill these destructive germs by heating them—the process we call pasteurization.

If germs could cause fermentation, Pasteur thought, perhaps they might cause infectious diseases as well. Eventually, that led him to confirm the germ theory of disease. It holds that pathogens such as viruses and bacteria, unseeable to the naked eye, invade human and animal hosts and give rise to infectious diseases. The acceptance of the germ theory would forever transform the practice of medicine, and the theory's link with the laboratory would confer on physicians the imprimatur of science. It remains the bedrock premise of modern medicine and medical research.

In the 1860s, Joseph Lister, a Glasgow surgeon, was an interested reader of Pasteur's, in particular a paper suggesting that heat, filtration, or exposure to chemicals might be used to kill the germs that caused gangrene. Lister tested this hypothesis by spraying carbolic acid on surgical instruments and incisions, thereby vastly reducing postoperative gangrene.

THE HISTORY OF INFECTION CONTROL

With the growing acceptance of the germ theory, hospitals increasingly used isolation to prevent the transmission of infectious diseases, and sanitary conditions in general improved, but hospitals continued to be breeding grounds for infection. Infectious diseases physicians and microbiologists gradually began to specialize in infection prevention, and a handful of hospitals developed infection control programs in the 1950s. Public health agencies initially kept their hands off, apparently believing that hospitals had the wherewithal to cure themselves, but in 1965, the Centers for Disease Control and Prevention (CDC) did make a major contribution to infection prevention with the creation of the Comprehensive Hospital Infections Project. Eight community hospitals around the United States were chosen to function as CDC laboratories for the study of healthcare-associated infection (HAI) epidemiology and the development of infection prevention techniques. The National Nosocomial Infections Surveillance System (NNIS) was established in 1970 to routinely collect hospital-acquired infection surveillance data for aggregation into a national database. In 2005, the CDC decided to combine the NNIS with the National Surveillance System for Healthcare Workers, a merger that included the Dialysis Surveillance Network, which the CDC had been separately managing under its Division of Healthcare Quality Promotion. Thus, the National Healthcare Safety Network (NHSN), a comprehensive system for the tracking of HAIs, was born. Starting with 300 hospitals, the network now gathers infection data from more than 11,000 medical facilities.

As infection control gained traction in hospitals, it became a potential new career path for staff members including nurses, microbiologists, and infectious diseases physicians, which, in turn, gave fresh impetus to the infection control movement. In 1972, they gained a professional society with the founding of the Association of Practitioners in Infection Control (APIC), now the Association for Professionals in Infection Control and Epidemiology, and other more specialized professional societies soon followed. These groups helped provide the trained professionals the infection prevention movement required to effectively reduce infections in U.S. hospitals.

Despite these signs of progress, the CDC was not satisfied with the state of HAI prevention. As a result, the agency initiated a national study in 1974 now known as the Study on the Effectiveness of Nosocomial Infection Control, or the SENIC Project. The study found that only about half of the 338 hospitals examined had infection surveillance and control systems, but those with such systems in place had substantially lower rates of HAI. That result convinced the Joint Commission on Accreditation of Hospitals to require, as of 1976, that hospitals must

operate CDC-recommended infection prevention programs to maintain their accreditation.

Yet HAI was still an afterthought when the Institute of Medicine published a watershed study in 1999 entitled, "To Err Is Human." It inspired
widespread media coverage, putting patient safety in general on the public
agenda, but it accorded HAI just five paragraphs—and even that in an
appendix to the main report. Infection prevention leaders, however, were
able to ride the patient safety wave, alerting the public to the extensive
and harmful impact of HAI. Their efforts led to the passage of state laws
requiring hospitals to publicly report their infection rates. The theory was
that this exposure of medical error would help spur hospitals to greater
efforts to prevent infection.

Since then, HAI has become a major component of the national and
international movement to enhance patient safety. Almost a third of the
hospital-acquired conditions that CMS no longer reimburses are HAIs.
About half of the initiatives in the Institute for Healthcare Improvement's
"100,000 Lives" campaign are concerned with infection prevention.

The infection prevention movement has come of age within the public health community. And our understanding of the technical side of
prevention has made great strides, which will become evident, we trust,
in the pages just ahead as we describe the bundles of interventions
behind catheter-associated urinary tract infection (CAUTI), central
line-associated bloodstream infection (CLABSI), and ventilator-associated
pneumonia (VAP) prevention. The greater challenge, the struggle to win
the active support of the clinical staff for these prevention initiatives, the
adaptive challenge, is described in the following chapters.

CAUTI

The popularity of the indwelling urinary catheter is impressive. More
than 100 million Foleys are used each year, worldwide, and U.S. hospitals account for more than a quarter of them. Foleys are often convenient,
for medical staff and for some patients. The use of an indwelling catheter

avoids the need for toileting patients, and requires only that the bag that collects urine be emptied when necessary.

Foleys are not, however, universally popular. One study[2] found that 42% of catheterized patients said the Foley was uncomfortable, 48% said it was painful, and 61% said it restricted their activities of daily living. It can serve as a one-point restraint, binding patients to their beds, which promotes such complications as venous thromboembolism and pressure ulcers. And if the Foley's balloon is not completely deflated upon removal, it can cause severe damage to the urinary tract. Catheterization can also delay patients' departure from a hospital if they cannot void normally following the Foley's removal.

The most important black mark against the Foley, though, is that it causes about 70% of all hospital-associated urinary tract infections. CAUTIs are one of the most common of all hospital infections. The longer the catheter remains in the body, the greater the chance that bacteria will travel up from the bag during routine maintenance of the Foley or any manipulation of the device.

At the model hospital we introduced in the previous chapter, the initiative to reduce CAUTI relies on a so-called bladder bundle, a combination of best practices, equipment, and protocols. Research by behavioral scientists has shown that the odds of success in infection control programs are improved by focusing on several modes of intervention rather than just one or two. That is not to say, however, that hospitals should take a multimodal-or-nothing approach; a more narrowly focused intervention is better than none.

The basic message of the bladder bundle is this: Don't use the Foley unless it's really necessary—and if you do use it, regularly reassess whether its use is still indicated and remove it as soon as possible.

The bundle at our model hospital includes:

- Hand hygiene: Use soap and water or an alcohol-based cleanser.
- A standardized kit containing a Foley with presealed junctions to prevent bacteria from entering the system, along with drapes

and other items to assure an aseptic insertion and proper
maintenance of the catheter.

- A urinary management policy that sets forth appropriate and
  inappropriate indications for the use of Foleys. Appropriate
  indications include acute urinary retention or bladder outlet
  obstruction; the need for accurate measurements of urinary
  output in critically ill patients; and a number of surgery-related
  circumstances. Inappropriate indications include using a Foley,
  instead of standard nursing practice, for urinary incontinence; for
  assessing urinary output in a patient who is not critically ill; and for
  obtaining urine for testing when the patient can voluntarily void.

- A standard operating procedure covering Foley insertion,
  maintenance, and removal. It calls for the use of a nursing
  assessment template added to the electronic medical record.
  Appropriate hand hygiene before and after handling the urinary
  catheter –à la Semmelweis—is also emphasized. Additionally, the
  protocol requires bedside nurses to make a daily template entry
  indicating whether any given Foley meets one or more of the
  appropriate indications for catheter use. If an in-place catheter
  fails that test, the nurse is to alert the appropriate physician
  caring for the patient and recommend the catheter's removal.
  Under a hospital protocol, nurses are empowered by a standing
  order to remove inappropriate Foleys if there is any substantial
  delay in obtaining the physician's agreement to the removal.

- A list of alternatives to the use of a Foley. They include intermittent
  catheterization with a straight catheter, a condom catheter in
  men, a portable bladder ultrasound to assess and manage urinary
  outflow, and other toileting options such as a bedpan or bedside
  commode.

The model hospital also employs two types of reminder systems. The first
simply alerts doctors and bedside nurses to the fact that a Foley is being
used by a patient and provides a list of the appropriate reasons to continue
or discontinue the catheter. The reminder (see Figure 3.1) is included in the

patient's chart and is part of the patient's electronic record. The model hospital, which uses computerized orders, also sends electronic reminders directly to the patient's physician. Reminders are generally dispatched as a hospital unit eases into an infection prevention initiative. Researchers have demonstrated the effectiveness of this reminder. One study[3] at a Veterans Health Administration medical center found that the use of a computerized reminder shortened the duration of catheterization by three days while not affecting the rate of recatheterization.

******* URINARY CATHETER REMINDER *******

Date: _____

This patient has had an indwelling urinary catheter since _____.

Please indicate below either your 1) approval to remove the catheter **OR**

2) state the reason for continued indwelling urinary catheterization.

- ☐ Please discontinue indwelling urinary catheter; **OR**

- ☐ Please continue indwelling urinary catheter because patient requires indwelling catheterization for the following reasons (please check all that apply):

  - ☐ Patient has acute urinary retention or bladder outlet obstruction

  - ☐ Need for accurate measurements of urinary output in critically ill patients

  - ☐ To assist in healing of open sacral or perineal wounds in incontinent patients

  - ☐ Patient requires prolonged immobilization (e.g., potentially unstable thoracic or lumbar spine, multiple traumatic injuriest such as pelvic fractures)

  - ☐ To improve comfort for end of life care if needed

  - ☐ Other- please specify: _____

_____   _____

Physician's Signature   Doctor Number

Figure 3.1
Example of a Urinary Catheter Reminder (adapted from Saint et al.[4] and Gould et al.[5])

The second type of reminder is the stop order, calling for the patient's bedside nurse to remove an unnecessary Foley. The model hospital is considering moving to a stop order that would prompt removal after 48 hours for both postoperative and medical patients if there no longer is an appropriate indication for the catheter to remain in place. Reminders of both varieties have proven their effectiveness. In one analysis of a number of CAUTI studies,[6] the reminders decreased infections by 53%.

CLABSI

In 1905, after considerable experimentation with dogs, Fritz Bleichröder, a Berlin physician and, incidentally, a son of Otto von Bismarck's banker, became the first person to perform a central venous catheterization on a human being. He decided not to publish his results at the time because he thought they had no practical value. He changed his mind several years later, and central venous catheterization went on to become a vital staple of modern medicine. The flexible catheter is threaded into a vein in the trunk of the body until it reaches a large vein near the heart, carrying nutrients, medicines, or blood, and it may remain in place for weeks on end.

For all its blessings, though, the central line can be dangerous or even deadly when bacteria grow in or around the device and move into the bloodstream. Each year, central line-associated bloodstream infection kills 12% to 25% of the more than 200,000 patients who develop it.

By the turn of the century, researchers had developed effective protocols to prevent CLABSI, but implementation was slow. In 2004, the nonprofit Institute for Healthcare Improvement launched its nationwide "100,000 Lives Campaign," which included CLABSI prevention as a specific target. The results were impressive. Between 2001 and 2009, the rate of CLABSI in intensive care units was reduced by 58%, achieving substantial human and financial benefits. In 2009, compared to 2001, up to 6,000 fewer lives were lost to CLABSI, and medical costs were cut by $414 million.[7]

Around the same time, the Keystone Center of the Michigan Health and Hospital Association launched the "Keystone ICU Initiative," which focused on the prevention of CLABSI in more than 100 ICUs across the state of Michigan. This federally funded and evidence-based intervention drastically reduced the mean rate of these infections per 1,000 catheter days from 7.7 infections at baseline to 1.4 infections 18 months later.[8] A similar intervention conducted at all 174 of the Veterans Health Administration's ICUs succeeded in cutting CLABSI rates from 3.8 per 1,000 catheter days in 2006 to 1.8 per 1,000 days in 2009.[9]

These achievements, however, were pretty much limited to the ICUs, where most of the prevention efforts have been focused. Today, 70% of patients with central lines are located outside the ICU, and the CLABSI incidence in these non-ICU units is sizable. As a result, more and more hospitals are developing initiatives tailored to control CLABSI beyond the ICU.

The central line most used outside the ICU does not start on its way toward the heart from the trunk of patients' bodies but from the arm. The peripherally inserted central catheter, or PICC, has a perceived lower complication rate than the traditional central line, and it allows patients to move around much more easily. The result: Far more than in the past, large numbers of sicker patients are being treated outside the ICU and many patients are even sent home with the PICC in place. For example, patients who need to be on an antibiotic for six weeks used to spend that time attached to a central line in the hospital; now, courtesy of the PICC, they are able to go home much sooner.

As is the case with the urinary catheter, the longer any device such as a central line stays in place, the greater the risk of infection. As a result, the CLABSI prevention bundle emphasizes the need to remove the catheter as soon as possible. The evidence-based CLABSI bundle—operationalized by using a checklist (see Box 3.1)—at our model hospital consists of:

- Hand hygiene: Use soap and water or an alcohol-based cleanser.
- Use maximum sterile barriers during insertion including mask, gloves, hair covering, sterile gown, and a sterile drape to cover the entire patient.

- Proper antiseptic: Use chlorhexidine gluconate to clean the skin when the catheter is inserted.
- Preferred veins: Avoid the femoral vein when possible.
- Daily review of each central line to determine whether it is still necessary, and prompt removal if it is not.

Box 3.1 **CENTRAL LINE INFECTION PREVENTION CHECKLIST (DEVELOPED BY PRONOVOST AND COL-LEAGUES[8] AND ADAPTED FROM GAWANDE[10])**

☑ Wash hands with soap before treating the patient.
☑ Clean the patient's skin with chlorohexidine antiseptic.
☑ Put sterile drapes over the entire patient.
☑ Wear a surgical mask, hat, sterile gown and gloves while carrying out the line insertion.
☑ Put a sterile dressing over the insertion site once the line is in.

At our model hospital, the chief medical officer, an intensivist herself, shows her support of the initiative by emphasizing the importance of using chlorhexidine rather than povidone-iodine as a skin cleanser. Each morning during rounds in the ICU, there is a routine discussion evaluating the necessity of all the lines in the unit, including central lines.

The usual central line insertion kit does not contain all the sterile barriers called for by the bundle. At the model hospital, the staff has worked with a manufacturer to develop an improved central line kit that contains all the necessary items. In the modified central line kit, chlorhexidine has been substituted for the traditional povidone-iodine and the small patient drape has been replaced by the required larger size drape that is used to ensure a maximum sterile barrier during central line insertion.

An infection preventionist at a hospital that adopted a similar approach told us about its impact: "It's becoming more and more difficult to not use [chlorhexidine rather than betadine] because that's what's available. People still have their stashes, it's a big hospital, but it's harder and harder."

When a central line is being inserted at the model hospital, the hospital protocol empowers nurses to stop the procedure if the bundle guidelines are not being followed. When that happens, a secondary goal is to avoid confrontation between nurse and physician.

At one of the hospitals we visited, a resident physician routinely neglected to wear a hat when she presided over a central line insertion. Finally, the nurse manager, holding a clipboard and pen, approached the doctor just before an insertion. "Let's see," the nurse said, "You're wearing a mask. O.K. Good. Let's see, were you going to wear a hat?" When the resident challenged her, the nurse replied, "I'm filling out this form for Dr. [Name of senior physician omitted]." "Wha . . . wha . . . Okay, gimme a hat," the resident said.

VAP

Ventilator-associated pneumonia strikes up to 20% of hospital patients on a ventilator for more than 48 hours. Their length of stay in the ICU is increased by up to a week and their length of stay in the hospital by up to 300%. Their risk of dying doubles.

The business end of the modern ventilator, the endotracheal tube, moves air directly in and out of the patient's lungs—most unlike the original 1928 breathing machine, the so-called iron lung, which achieved its goal indirectly. The patient, usually a victim of paralytic polio, lay in the metal chamber while a pump removed the air, lowering the air pressure and enabling the lungs to expand and the patient to breathe.

The immediate precursor of today's ventilator appeared in World War II, and used positive air pressure; delivered through facemasks, it allowed fighter pilots to operate at ever-higher altitudes. Endotracheal tubes began to appear in hospitals in the 1950s, both as a better treatment for polio patients and as a result of the increased use of muscle relaxants during anesthesia. Although the relaxants improved operating conditions, they also paralyzed the patient, requiring mechanical ventilation. The endotracheal tubes are also used on ICU patients who need sedation or are suffering acute respiratory failure.

For all its benefits, the tube can easily become a host for bacteria that cause pneumonia. That can happen when patients cough, aspirating food particles that lodge in the tube, and when saliva and mucus build up on the tube's outside rim. By following the instructions of the evidence-based VAP bundle, hospitals can greatly minimize the pneumonia risk. As was the case with CAUTI and CLABSI, the best safeguard against infection is the prompt removal of the tube. At the model hospital, the VAP bundle's instructions are reproduced on the patient's electronic medical record and paper chart.

- Interrupt the delivery of sedatives, otherwise known as sedation vacation, on a daily basis. This will determine the patient's readiness to stop ventilation. One study[11] showed that sedation vacations shortened ventilation by an average of more than two days and cut patients' stay in the ICU by 3.5 days.
- Elevate the head of the patient's bed by 30 degrees to 45 degrees, reducing the likelihood of aspiration. Judging the degree of elevation can be a problem. "The nurses thought that they were already putting the head of the bed up 30 degrees," an ICU nurse told us, "but if you looked at the angle of the bed, it was only 20."
- Clean out the patient's mouth with chlorhexidine daily to clear away bacteria.
- Cease mechanical ventilation as soon as possible.

Physicians today have an increasingly popular alternative to the endotracheal tube for patients who are unable to breathe normally because of the use of muscle relaxants during surgery or some other cause—noninvasive positive-pressure ventilation (NPPV). The move toward ventilation without an artificial airway had its start in the 1980s when physicians began prescribing continuous positive airway pressure (CPAP) via a nasal mask for those with sleep apnea. A decade later, that approach was tried out for the treatment of such ailments as congestive heart failure and postoperative respiratory failure, and it has since become a first-line therapy in some major hospitals.

NPPV has two basic modes, continuous positive pressure for the patient who is breathing spontaneously and bilevel positive airway pressure (BiPAP), which delivers both inspiratory and expiratory positive airway pressure, for the patient with respiratory failure. The air passes through a face mask, a nasal mask, or a helmet that covers the head.

For patients, NPPV represents a far more comfortable option as compared to the endotracheal tube—and it virtually banishes the risk of pneumonia that is associated with the tube.

WHEN PROOF IS HARD TO FIND

The medical community has achieved amazing progress in the battle against disease, in part because of the development of advanced devices like NPPV and new types of skin disinfectants. Each of these practices must prove itself clinically as we discover its pros and cons and learn to ignore or cope with unforeseen complications. Over time, one generation gives way to the next, the new piece of equipment correcting previous complications and inevitably introducing new ones.

New devices, much as the items in the quality improvement bundles we have been describing, win medical acceptance in part because of their scientific backing. The gold standard in such matters, of course, is the randomized controlled trial in which the study subjects are randomly assigned to one treatment group or the other. It's a high, and frequently unattainable, standard for quality initiatives. A 2003 tongue-in-cheek exploration of the limits of the randomized trial, published in the *British Medical Journal*, addresses the problem. A proper study of parachutes' effectiveness "in preventing major trauma related to gravitational challenge," the authors point out, would require that a random set of individuals jump from a height without parachutes. Our experience of life leads us to be confident about preferring parachutes to a free fall, but where's the proof?[12]

There have been evidence-based studies showing that the longer a Foley remains in a patient, the greater the likelihood of infection. However, a randomized controlled trial of the CAUTI bundle would be difficult, since it would require hospitals to withhold appropriate management from ill patients. Rather, the CAUTI prevention bladder bundle is a best practice approach, approved by the medical community as a whole. It is also a collection of items with a range of scientific support. There is stronger evidence for those items that speak directly to the Foley's length of stay in a patient, for instance, than for those that require aseptic insertion (as opposed to "clean" insertion).

This discrepancy in scientific backing among elements of an infection bundle is echoed in comparisons among prevention bundles. The evidence for the CLABSI bundle, for instance, is considerably stronger than for its CAUTI counterpart. These differences in proof can help decide how a prevention bundle is received by nurses and physicians—it's one reason that hospitals overall have welcomed CLABSI prevention efforts more than CAUTI prevention.

In the next chapter, we move from the specific devices and technical practices of infection prevention to focus on the adaptive side. We return to the model hospital to see how our CAUTI project manager goes about selecting her team—and how they prepare for the all-important task of implementation. Their ability to predict and find solutions for the personal and institutional roadblocks ahead will decide the fate of the initiative.

SUGGESTIONS FOR FURTHER READING

Gawande, A. (December 10, 2007). The checklist: If something so simple can transform intensive care, what else can it do? New Yorker, 10, 86–101.

　　In his engaging and thought-provoking style, Gawande discusses the modern challenges facing intensive care units and their staff. Using the work of Peter

Pronovost, MD, PhD, and the successful results of the central line checklist he implemented first at Johns Hopkins Hospital and later throughout the state of Michigan, Gawande explores the complexity of caring for the sickest patients given the multitude of opportunities to introduce error.

Gould, C. V., Umscheid, C. A., Agarwal, R. K., Kuntz, G., Pegues, D. A., & Healthcare Infection Control Practices Advisory Committee. (2010). Guidelines for prevention of catheter-associated urinary tract infections 2009. *Infection Control and Hospital Epidemiology, 31*(4), 319–326.

This guide both updates and expands the original Centers for Disease Control and Prevention's guidelines for prevention of catheter-associated urinary tract infections from 1981. This edition, often referred to as the "HICPAC Guidelines," provides examples of appropriate and inappropriate indications for indwelling urethral catheter use and was developed using a targeted, systematic review of the best available evidence, though their final indications are based primarily on expert consensus.

Lo, E., Nicolle, L., Coffin, S. E., Gould, C., Maragakis, l., Meddings, J., . . . Yokoe, D. S. (2014). Strategies to prevent catheter-associated urinary tract infections in acute care hospitals. *Infection Control and Hospital Epidemiology, 35*(5), 464–479.

In this compendium, the authors highlight some of the practical recommendations for acute care hospitals in their efforts to prevent catheter-associated urinary tract infection. Using the most up-to-date evidence and presented in a concise format, strategies for CAUTI detection, prevention, and performance measures are reviewed.

Marschall, J., Mermel, L. A., Fakih, M., Hadaway, L., Kallen, A., O'Grady, N. P., . . . Yokoe, D. S. (2014). Strategies to prevent central line-associated bloodstream infections in acute care hospitals. *Infection Control and Hospital Epidemiology, 35*(7), 753–771.

As with the catheter-associated urinary tract infection compendium, the authors update the previously published guidelines for central line-associated bloodstream infection prevention in acute care hospitals. Using the most up-to-date evidence and presented in a concise format, strategies for CLABSI detection, prevention, and performance measures are reviewed.

O'Grady, N. P., Alexander, M., Burns, L. A., Dellinger, E. P., Garland, J., Heard, S. O., . . . the Healthcare Infection Control Practices Advisory Committee. (2011). Summary of recommendations: Guidelines for the prevention of intravascular catheter-related infections. *Clinical Infectious Diseases, 52*(9), 1087–1099.

This report, prepared by a multidisciplinary working group in collaboration with more than 15 professional societies, replaces the 2002 Guideline for Prevention of Intravascular Catheter-Related Infections. Each of the recommendations is categorized based on the strength of existing scientific data, theoretical rationale, applicability, and economic impact.

Pittet, D., Hugonnet, S., Harbarth, S., Mourouga, P., Sauvan, V., Touveneau, S. & Perneger, T.V. (2000). Effectiveness of a hospital-wide programme to improve compliance with hand hygiene. *The Lancet, 356*(9238), 1307–1312.

In this observational study, Pittet and colleagues monitored the overall compliance with hand hygiene during routine patient care in a teaching hospital in Geneva, Switzerland, before and during implementation of a hand hygiene campaign. The authors found that compliance improved from 48% in 1994 to 66% in 1997 ($p < 0.001$), overall nosocomial infection decreased (prevalence of 16.9% in 1994 to 9.9% in 1998; $p = 0.04$), MRSA transmission rates decreased (2.16 to 0.93 episodes per 10,000 patient-days; $p < 0.001$), and the consumption of alcohol-based handrub solution increased from 3.5 to 15.4 L per 1,000 patient-days between 1993 and 1998 ($p < 0.001$).

Rotter, M. L. (1998). Semmelweis' sesquicentennial: A little noted anniversary of handwashing. *Current Opinion in Infectious Diseases, 11*(4), 457–460.

This review describes Hungarian obstetrician Ignaz Philipp Semmelweis's achievements from 150 years ago. In addition to documenting Semmelweis's observation of the importance of hand hygiene in disease prevention, Rotter discusses the current lack of compliance by some health professionals and concludes that 150 years later, hand hygiene "still remains an educational problem to be solved."

Building the Team

Never doubt that a small group of thoughtful, concerned citizens can change the world. Indeed it is the only thing that ever has.

—MARGARET MEAD

"Surgeons are very tribal," the chief of staff said, discussing the difficulty that an infection prevention leader might have trying to bring his message to a group of surgeons. "The first thing we're going to do is we're going to say, 'Look, you're not one of us.' The way to get buy-in from surgeons is you got to have a surgeon on your team."

A successful infection prevention initiative requires, above all, highly motivated and effective team members, and a maximum of forward planning. The project manager, the nurse and physician champions, and any other team members need to think long and hard about the problems they are likely to face in pursuing the initiative. They need to search, ahead of time, for ways to confront or avoid those problems, such as corralling a surgeon for the team.

The team's primary goal is to create what is, in effect, a "people bundle," the adaptive counterpart to the technical focus of the bladder bundle. Too often, in the effort to effect change and implement best practices, short shrift is given to the "people" aspect of the process. It takes a village, the widespread cooperation of a hospital's nurses and doctors, to secure a successful quality initiative. And it takes an organized, intensive team effort, implementing a people bundle, to gain that cooperation.

At our model hospital, building a team is the new project manager's first order of business. Why the team approach? Why not just a letter from the hospital's chief executive officer or chief medical officer announcing a new safety initiative: "From this day forward, all bedside nurses will fill out a checklist at shift's end reporting on the presence of Foleys in their units and will ask physicians to remove unnecessary catheters"? Because it doesn't work. Note the effect of hospitals' continuing insistence that all their healthcare workers must have a yearly flu vaccination: a nationwide response rate of just 67% for the 2011–2012 season.[1] It takes more than a C-suite command to convince bedside nurses to adopt an operational change that will add to their already substantial workload.

In this chapter, we describe the team recruiting process for a medical floor-based intervention at the midsize, 250-bed model hospital. The personnel and structure of a team will generally vary with the size of the facility. At a small hospital, the team might consist of just the project manager and a nurse champion, since the number of patients with indwelling urinary catheters is typically no more than a handful. A large hospital might have a process improvement team already in place and ready to take on any safety initiative. The creation of a project team will also vary somewhat depending on what part of the hospital is to be targeted—the medical floor, as here, or the operating room or emergency department, where the vast majority of Foleys are inserted. (More on that topic later in the chapter.)

RECRUITING A NURSE CHAMPION

The nurse champion at our model hospital will most likely be a nurse unit manager, a charge nurse, a nurse educator, or a staff nurse. She needs to know her way around the hospital hierarchy, but be independent-minded in terms of finding solutions. She should have a strong commitment to patient safety. And she must be on good terms with her colleagues. By way of contrast, when a nurse executive or director of nursing becomes nurse champion, there is the danger that the bedside nurses will view the infection prevention initiative as just another occasion for obeying the boss, rather than as a nurse-based effort to better serve patients. Far more than the physician champion, the nurse champion will be the embodiment of the project to the people who will decide its fate: the bedside nurses.

In fact, given the right set of circumstances, a bedside nurse can be a formidable nurse champion. We know of one example of that arrangement—a bedside nurse who attended planning meetings as well as the monthly meetings post-implementation on her own time, and whose dedication to infection prevention became, well, contagious among her colleagues throughout the hospital.

The potential nurse champion will, inevitably, be a busy person. To win her participation, the project manager at the model hospital begins by assuring her that she will be given time off to attend planning and reporting sessions, and that she will be able to handle other project duties during her regular shifts. The manager makes it clear that the nurse champion will be a full partner in the infection prevention enterprise and that the project will have the full support of the hospital leadership and other staff members; that includes case managers, who equate reduced complications with lower costs, and who understand that the early removal of a catheter can reduce a patient's length of stay. Infection preventionists will be in her corner not only because the bladder bundle can reduce urinary tract infection, but also because it can cut back on antimicrobial use.

The project manager also lets the potential nurse champion know that her work will be recognized in her annual evaluation appraisals, and in communications with the chief nursing officer. Her efforts may also be publicly acknowledged in a hospital newsletter or with a "nurse champion award" presented during a hospital town hall meeting or other staff recognition event. Above all, the manager appeals to the nurse's concern for the comfort and safety of her patients—the concern that inspired her career to begin with and is the primary force behind the intervention.

ENLISTING A PHYSICIAN CHAMPION

To enlist a physician champion, the project manager will look among the hospital epidemiologists, hospitalists, infectious diseases specialists, and those whose specialty is relevant to the particular infection prevention target, urologists in this case. She wants a physician who has pride in the hospital's culture of excellence, or concern over the lack of one. She seeks a person who has the ear of the hospital administration and the respect of his or her peers, a doctors' doctor, and someone who has the patience to hear out people who disagree with his or her point of view. The search for volunteers is complicated by the fact that some of the doctors are not employees of the hospital. As private practitioners, they may lack a sense of identification with the facility and they are comparatively free of its authority. Convincing any physician, employee, or nonemployee, to take on extra work beyond his current practice is likely to be a tough assignment.

Some hospitals have experimented with giving employee physicians a financial bonus to shoulder quality improvement roles, but, as one medical director told us, that's "kind of a slippery slope." Paying doctors to take part in a patient-centered intervention seems inappropriate to us. We see no problem, though, with temporarily relieving the physician of some of his responsibilities or, as was done in one hospital, recognizing a member of the medical staff with a "physician champion" award, complete with a certificate signed by the hospital's chief of staff and a gift certificate to a local restaurant.

In her discussions with potential physician champions, the project manager at the model hospital emphasizes the need to take action against infection, in general, and in this hospital, in particular. She emphasizes that the project's protocols are reliable, straight from the Centers for Disease Control and Prevention (CDC), and offers examples of successful infection prevention interventions in nearby facilities. She informs these physicians that the hospital administration has given the project a high priority, and that she and the administration view doctors as full partners in the project, not as barriers. She cites the medical reasons why physician champions can count on the support of their colleagues—rehabilitation specialists and geriatricians, for example—because Foleys reduce patient mobility, and urologists because the insertion and removal of the devices can lead to urethral damage and other patient-related injuries. Early and often, she assures physicians that the champion role will not take too much of their time. They will not, for instance, be expected to attend all meetings or be otherwise involved in matters unrelated to clinical concerns, such as budget discussions or internal promotion plans or working out details of data collection, unless, of course, they want to be. Their chief responsibility will be to share the details of the intervention with colleagues and gain their cooperation.

In making her team selections, the project manager needs to avoid choosing people on the basis of their job title. Unfortunately, titles don't guarantee that a person will be appropriate for this task. Case in point: For an intervention to prevent healthcare-associated infection (HAI), the infection preventionist might seem like an obvious choice for project manager. And we have, indeed, encountered some infection preventionists who were perfect for this task because they were on cordial terms with everyone in their hospitals, doctors and nurses alike; cared deeply about the intervention; and knew just what buttons to push to keep a project on track. But we also found others who were fixated on surveillance and infection rates and were not well versed in the behavioral changes necessary to ensure a successful intervention.

Hospitalists are also seemingly natural members or leaders of the project team. These physicians, who now number 30,000 in the United States alone, spend their days in the hospital, interacting with nurses and patients. They tend to be considerably younger than most other physicians in the hospital with more of a team-centered approach to medicine and thus may have far better relationships with nurses. But because their age could be a handicap in dealing with older doctors, hospitalists may sometimes not be ideal for leadership roles in an intervention.

The project manager also needs to beware of the tendency to choose from the same pool of people who always seem to get tapped to lead quality improvement projects. They tend to be overcommitted and thus unable to devote the necessary time and energy to any one given initiative.

Aside from the project manager and the nurse and physician champions, the team will generally include someone to handle data, typically an infection preventionist, or a member of the quality improvement department. He or she will collate information—specifically, the presence of a Foley, the explanation for its original insertion or continued use, and any indication of a healthcare-associated urinary tract infection—and feed it back to the floor unit involved and to the hospital office responsible for sending the results to the CDC. (See Figure 4.1.) The addition of other team members may be delayed until after the team has selected the medical unit that will be the campaign's first target, in order to bring in people who will be close to the action.

The executive sponsor is an ex-officio member of the team. She sits down with the project manager every two weeks to monitor the intervention's progress, and makes an occasional, unannounced appearance at meetings. She expects that the project manager will clear major decisions with her. The sponsor wants the team as a whole to understand that

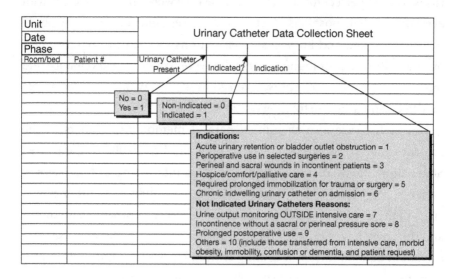

Figure 4.1
Example Urinary Catheter Data Collection Sheet.

she represents the hospital leadership's continuing interest in the initiative, and that she is there for them if a need arises, though she has every confidence that they will handle this assignment on their own with flying colors. (See Table 4.1.)

HOW THE TEAM OPERATES

In a quality improvement initiative, as in so many of life's endeavors, nothing succeeds like success. For the team at the model hospital to convince administrators and medical leaders that the infection prevention intervention is effective, and worth introducing throughout the institution, clear proof will be required. This is how the team plans to go about it.

The intervention will start small, with a single 20-bed unit, so that the team can easily monitor results and quickly resolve any problems that crop up during the implementation phase. The project manager is looking for a unit that has a track record of cooperating with earlier quality initiatives— there's no need to look for trouble—but is not in the midst of too many at the moment. The unit should also have a full share of Foleys in place as well as a high rate of catheter-associated urinary tract infection (CAUTI), so that the campaign improvement will be as impressive as possible.

After consulting with nursing staff familiar with the individual medical floor units, the team will choose three or four such units. The project manager will then arrange for the collection of key data from each of those units over a five-day period: the presence of a Foley, the explanation for its original insertion, and why it is currently still in place. In addition, information about the CAUTI rates for the units will be obtained from the infection preventionist. This baseline data hopefully will, when compared to data collected during and after implementation of the initiative, provide the proof needed to convince administration and clinical leaders to expand the campaign to other parts of the hospital. It will also determine which of the several units under consideration is best suited to be the campaign's first target.

TABLE 4.1 AN EXAMPLE OF THE ROLES & RESPONSIBILITIES OF THE MEMBERS OF A TEAM (ADAPTED FROM FAKIH ET AL.[2])

Role or responsibility	Example of personnel to consider, and some advice
Project coordinator/ team manager	Infection preventionist, quality manager, nurse manager *When selecting a team leader, consider whether the team leader has successfully led another quality improvement project. Generally the leadership skills and previous success are more important than the job title or content expertise.*
Nurse champion	Nurse manager, charge nurse, staff nurse, nurse educator *For a CAUTI prevention initiative, if you do not already have a nurse champion, consider a charge nurse or nurse manager rather than a bedside nurse. They generally have more time away from the bedside and are thus able to help with other initiatives. In addition, they generally have more influence over other nurses. This person is needed to obtain buy-in from other nurses because often these CAUTI initiatives can involve additional nursing effort (monitoring indwelling urinary catheter placement, monitoring indications, more time toileting patients, and possible involvement in data collection).*
Physician champion	Hospitalist, hospital epidemiologist, infectious diseases specialist, geriatrician, emergency physician, urologist *A physician champion can be key to the success of the initiative. Try to involve a physician who is highly regarded or has the ear of other physicians. If you do not have access to a physician who is willing to be an actively involved physician champion, then consider selecting a respected physician who is willing to lend his or her name to this initiative without doing most of the actual work.*
Data collection, monitoring, and reporting	Infection preventionist, quality manager, patient safety officer *For a CAUTI prevention initiative, someone must be responsible for collecting data on CAUTI outcomes and indwelling urinary catheter prevalence. This can be the same person who currently collects these data for the hospital.*

The First Meeting

To open the first formal meeting of the team, which may also be attended by other interested hospital personnel, the project manager presents a larger vision of the intervention. Hospital infections are a national problem, she says, and it's a serious problem in this hospital. The CEO is very concerned. But then the project manager switches gears: She speaks of the needless human pain caused by CAUTI. She tells stories of real patients who developed CAUTI and the suffering they endured, as well as the noninfectious complications that accompany use of the Foley. Her message: This project is not simply another bureaucratic exercise, and it is not simply another research project dreamed up by academics; it is crucially important for the hospital and for its patients.

At the meeting, the project manager shares the published literature of what others have done to reduce the incidence of CAUTI and shows a video describing the components of the bladder bundle. The nurse champion answers any clinical questions attendees may have about the actual insertion and removal of the Foley as currently practiced in the hospital, and explains the various alternatives to the indwelling catheter. The project manager then walks her listeners through the plans for the implementation process, rehearsing the various steps along the way, including her determination not to start the intervention during the summer vacation season. She solicits suggestions and clarifications.

An infection preventionist asks whether a computer-based self-learning module has been considered as a way to educate bedside nurses and physicians in the details of the bladder bundle. She says one had been used to good effect at the hospital where she had previously worked. The module explained the connection between Foleys and CAUTI and included directions for the proper placement and maintenance of the catheters. Those assigned to use the module were given a date for completion after which their understanding of the material was evaluated. The one thing the module lacked, she says, was sufficient emphasis on communicating the requirements of the bladder bundle to physicians. The project manager says that a self-learning module might be a good possibility if the intervention extends to the whole hospital.

The project manager is reminded of another computer-based, interactive program, this one developed by the U.S. Department of Health and Human Services. It presents dramatized scenarios related to healthcare-associated infection prevention and gives clinicians a chance to "play it out before you live it out." The problem, she points out, is that the program is focused on other infections, not CAUTI.[3]

A nurse supervisor recalls encountering a real-life version of the agency's approach at a meeting devoted to improving nurse-physician relations. The nurses and doctors at the session took turns going through likely scenarios, a physician giving an inappropriate order for a Foley, for example, or a nurse asking a physician for an order to remove a catheter from a patient.

The project manager has finished drafting a new version of the hospital's CAUTI prevention policy and procedures to reflect the components of the bladder bundle. At the meeting, she passes around a copy of the draft, seeking feedback from the other team members. A nurse suggests that the draft should include having a nurse who is trained in the new catheter policy take part in daily rounds. That sets off a lively debate, which the project manager finally cuts off, pleading time pressures. She says she will raise the possibility verbally when she submits her draft to the project's executive sponsor, but cautions that the leadership is unlikely to be ready to take that step.

She then outlines her plans for promoting the intervention within the hospital, building hospital-wide support for the day when the campaign spreads to other units including the emergency department and intensive care units. Educational posters will be hung in high-traffic spots such as nursing lounges and restrooms and flyers distributed, proclaiming, "Get That Urinary Catheter Out!" and "Ex-Foley-Ate." Space will be set aside on the hospital's website and in its newsletters for a description of healthcare-associated infection and an announcement of the new initiative to deal with it. Campaign messages will also be regularly broadcast on social networks such as Facebook and Twitter.

But the most important promotion, the project manager insists, is the one that team members and their supporters will undertake in their daily contacts with hospital staff: the physicians in their conversations with colleagues and in presentations at grand rounds or at medical staff conferences; the nurses at morning report, in-service training, and in one-on-one talks. And she urges them to use, where feasible, their own version of the emotional appeal with which she started the meeting, to put a human face on the campaign. Convincing nurses and doctors to revise long-time routine procedures and winning their acceptance of a change in the nurse-doctor relationship along the way—all that, the project manager admits, is a tall order. It will take all of the team's persuasive powers, she warns. And that process should start ASAP.

The project manager also reports that three units have been chosen as potential candidates to be the initial target of the initiative. She says she has initiated the collection of baseline data from these units, and she promises to identify the ultimate target unit at the next meeting.

The Follow-Up

Ten days later, the project manager is as good as her word: She starts the follow-up meeting by announcing that the initiative will focus first on 4 West, a 20-bed unit with the best combination of willing nurses and indwelling urinary catheters. The nurse champion is already bringing the unit's nurse educator up to speed on the bladder bundle to help prepare her for her sessions explaining the intervention to the unit's bedside nurses. The rest of the meeting is devoted to rehearsing the implementation of the bladder bundle, making sure there is a standard operating procedure in place, and discussing potential problems. Does the unit have enough intermittent straight catheters on hand? Is there a portable bladder scanner on the unit? Are there other quality improvement activities underway or scheduled on 4 West that need to be coordinated with? Are there personal traits or quirks of the 4 West leadership that the team needs to watch out for? Will the nursing staff get with the program? Have the elements of the bundle been properly integrated into the patient record system?

The start of the implementation is scheduled for the following Monday. On Sunday, both the day and night nursing staffs receive text messages reminding them of the event. But there is no celebration—no ribbon cutting, no bagels—on Monday morning. This is not the first quality improvement program the unit has undertaken, nor will it be the last, and the staff has other fish to fry—catching up on weekend developments, for example.

But the executive sponsor does show up at the unit's morning meeting to emphasize the importance of the intervention. The nurse champion is there as well, and she will visit the unit most days during initial implementation, checking in with the unit manager and chatting with one or another of the nurses to see how the project is going. But it will be the task of the unit manager and the charge nurse to make sure the bedside nurses understand and are performing their key role in the project.

At least once a day, the nurses of 4 West are to become the Foley Police, or catheter patrol, as many hospitals have dubbed them. They note on the Foley template on the computerized patient record system whether their patients have an indwelling catheter; if the device is newly inserted, the reason for its placement; and otherwise the reason that it is still in place. And, if there is not an appropriate reason for the catheter, according to the bladder bundle, the nurses are to inform the physician and suggest the removal of the Foley. That's the theory, but as will be seen in Chapter 6, there can be a formidable chasm between theory and practice.

If the intervention succeeds on 4 West, if the use of Foleys decreases substantially and the infection rate drops, the campaign is scheduled to move on to other units and, eventually, to the emergency department and intensive care units. The challenges will be substantial on the wards, since each unit has its own personality, and its variety of personalities, but the basic mode of operation is similar from one unit to the next. The emergency department and intensive care units represent very different environments, compared to the medical floor and to each other. So as the campaign expands, the personnel of the project team will inevitably change to match the new target sites.

PREVENTING CAUTI IN THE EMERGENCY DEPARTMENT

The key to a successful CAUTI prevention initiative in an emergency department (ED) is the active participation of one or more emergency medicine physicians.[4] In that hectic and unpredictable environment, the physicians and nurses properly see themselves as serving on the front lines. As an ED chief put it, "When you are working in the pit, and see it the way we do, having one of us carry the ball brings a level of credibility to the table that outside physicians don't exactly bring." Nurses and doctors are more concerned about whether their patients are still breathing than about whether they have a catheter. It takes a member of the team to convince the ED that catheters count.

Traditionally, indwelling catheters are placed automatically in ED patients with severe enough problems to require them to stay on in the hospital, and the nurses don't want them walking around. When the patients are ready to leave for the wards, the nurses seldom pause to remove the Foleys, which explains why most indwelling catheters on the medical wards come from the ED.

So the first goal of the bladder bundle's project manager in the ED is to convince physicians and nurses to make sure a patient's condition warrants an indwelling catheter, and to consider safer alternatives such as a condom catheter, or a bladder scanner with intermittent straight catheterization. The second goal is to convince them to have the Foleys removed, where appropriate, before the patients move to the medical floor. (At some hospitals, ED nurses said they left in catheters as a favor to the floor nurses, to save them the trouble of reinserting.)

The project leader can demonstrate the importance of the intervention by sharing with her team the latest data from the medical floor, in particular figures showing how many of the floor's Foleys started out in the ED and what percentage of them led to an infection. He can call a meeting of physicians to seek their cooperation in the initiative. The most effective approach, though, is for him and/or the nurse champion to spend a part of each day walking through the department, reminding everyone they see about the intervention, asking a nurse or a physician whether that Foley they are about to insert is really necessary, whether it meets the appropriateness criteria. Or asking whether the patient being rolled toward the entrance to the wards has a Foley in place, and whether it's still needed. "It took a while," one ED chief said, "but eventually they got the message, and they did not want to see us anymore. They knew their old habits were probably not best for the patient."

PREVENTING CAUTI IN THE INTENSIVE CARE UNIT

The intensive care unit (ICU) has its own team spirit, rooted in a feeling that it is a special place—the life-saving arm of the hospital—and it takes a team member to lead a successful initiative there. Project managers have their work cut out for them: As in the ED, the default position is to insert Foleys. In a unit whose nurses spend their days monitoring patients' symptoms on a maze of machines, interrupted by intermittent crises, the indwelling urinary catheter offers a touch of simplicity, an easy way to keep track of a patient's intake and urinary output. Of course, for seriously ill patients who need their urine output monitored by the hour, Foleys are clearly desirable. These patients will receive medications and fluids based on urine output measurements. But for many other critical care patients, especially those from the operating room, the goal is, in fact, to get them up and walking as soon as possible and having a Foley can delay that result.

Patients' stay in the ED is measured in hours, whereas intensive care patients typically spend several days there. That greatly increases the odds that a Foley, whether appropriately or inappropriately inserted, has outlived its time and should be removed. Project managers need to see that "presence/rationale for Foley" is added to the daily checklists and "discontinue Foley" is added to the postoperative order sets.

Bladder bundle interventions have generally not devoted much time and energy to converting operating room personnel. When a surgery is going to run on for six hours or so, the indwelling catheter is a logical option. Shorter procedures are questionable in that regard, but many surgical personnel automatically and insistently use Foleys.

We were told of an orthopedic procedure that was scheduled to last a few hours. When a nurse prepared to insert a Foley, an observer familiar with the bladder bundle philosophy suggested that the catheter was not necessary. The anesthesiologist protested. He wanted that Foley, he said, because he didn't want to have to worry about urinary retention—he had enough other things to think about. He did not welcome the suggestion that CAUTI was also worth worrying about.

In the next chapter, we discuss the role of quality improvement leadership in the C-suite and among project managers and team champions. Topics include the varieties of leadership approaches and the power of emotional intelligence.

SUGGESTED FURTHER READING

Collins, J. (2001). *Good to great: Why some companies make the leap. . . and others don't.* New York, NY: HarperBusiness.

> Setting out to answer the question, "Can a good company become great?" this book looks in depth at 11 companies that made substantial improvements in their performance over time to see if there were any common traits among them. What the author discovered challenged much of the conventional wisdom of the time.

Damschroder, L. J., Banaszak-Holl, J., Kowalski, C. P., Forman, J., Saint, S., & Krein, S. L. (2009). The role of the champion in infection prevention: Results from a multisite qualitative study. *Quality and Safety in Health Care, 18*(6), 434–440.

> In this multisite, mixed-methods study of 86 individuals (14 VA and non-VA hospitals), Damschroder and colleagues explored the types and numbers of champions who led efforts to implement best practices to prevent healthcare-associated infection in U.S. hospitals. Their findings suggest that the factors that influence the choice of champions vary with the type of practice implemented (new technology versus behavior changes) and that the quality of the organizational networks affects the effectiveness of the champions.

Fakih, M. G., Pena, M. E., Shemes, S., Rey, J., Berriel-Cass, D., Szpunar, S. M., Savoy-Moore, R. T., & Saravolatz, L. D. (2010). Effect of establishing guidelines on appropriate urinary catheter placement. *Academic Emergency Medicine, 17*(3), 337–340.

> In this study, the authors sought to evaluate the effect of establishing institutional guidelines for appropriate urinary catheter placement and physician education in

the emergency department of their academic medical center. They found that 15% of patients had urinary catheters placed, but only 47% of those insertions had a physician's order documented (of those documented, 75.5% were appropriately indicated compared to 52% when no documentation was present). These results indicate that establishing guidelines for urinary catheter placement and physician education in the emergency department was associated with a marked reduction in utilization.

The Importance of Leadership and Followership

My own definition of leadership is this: The capacity and the will to rally men and women to a common purpose and the character which inspires confidence.

—GENERAL BERNARD MONTGOMERY

Each year, the American College of Healthcare Executives surveys hospital CEOs to see what's worrying them the most. Their top concern in 2012 was all too familiar: "Financial challenges" has held top ranking for years. The surprise was number two: "Patient safety and quality" displaced "healthcare reform implementation," which had held second place since its introduction to the survey in 2009.[1]

Did that mean CEOs were spending more time on quality improvement, such as preventing healthcare-associated infection? Not according to the 2013 returns, which showed "patient safety" kicked back to a third-place tie with "government mandates," whereas "financial challenges" and "healthcare reform" were back at numbers one and two. Too bad. The C-suite has an important role in the kind of initiatives described in these pages.

In our studies of quality improvement interventions, we found a siz-able number of top leaders who devoted considerable time and energy to promoting these initiatives. At one hospital, an infection preventionist reported that "several of our vice presidents. . . would actually go to the units and talk with the staff and see how [the initiative] was going."

On the other hand, we discovered hospitals that had completed very successful projects to reduce central line-associated bloodstream infec-tion (CLABSI) and catheter-associated urinary tract infection (CAUTI) whose top executives did nothing more for the projects than refrain from rejecting them. The leadership came from elsewhere in the institution, from physicians and nurses in every department and on every bureau-cratic level.

NONPROFITS ARE DIFFERENT

Surprisingly little has been written, in the popular media or in academe, about leadership in a hospital setting. There has been a general assumption that the best practices of leadership in business can be directly applied to nonprofit institutions. Our research suggests otherwise, and we find that view supported by the business consultant and author Jim Collins. In a monograph entitled *Good to Great and the Social Sectors* he contrasts the goals of the two worlds: "In the social sectors, the critical question is not, 'How much money do we make per dollar of invested capital?' but, 'How effectively do we deliver on our mission and make a distinctive impact, relative to our resources?' "[2]

That divergence has led to substantially different management struc-tures and roles. In for-profit corporations, the CEO possesses the power to make decisions, on his own if that's his style, confident that his hierar-chy will implement them. His leadership tends to be transactional, ensur-ing that employee roles are clearly delineated and motivating employees with punishments and rewards. But in such institutions as universities, charities, and hospitals, the CEO and his or her top aides must cope with a variety of independent power bases—tenured professors, volunteers, physicians—who generally don't do well at taking orders. The result, Collins says: Two distinct kinds of leadership approaches. For-profit leaders in general exercise executive, command-and-control skills, whereas social sector leaders, if they want to succeed, must learn legislative skills such as the ability to communicate, listen, and persuade. Their leadership tends to be transformational rather than transactional, inspiring personnel to see beyond their immediate self-interest.[3] (See Box 5.1.)

The most successful hospital leaders, for example, are ambitious not so much for themselves or for the bottom line, Collins suggests, but for the institution's patient-centered mission. To effectively lead physicians, nurses, and other personnel who have a major personal stake in their life-saving profession, a leader, whatever her title, must share that motivation. The transformational leader adapts to the needs and motives of her followers and seeks to earn their trust. With their willing support, she can draw on the individual expertise and imagination so necessary to reaching and implementing the right decisions.

In his monograph, Collins describes a meeting he had with a group of nonprofit healthcare leaders. As he had found in so many social sector sessions, the healthcare people obsessed about systemic constraints.

Box 5.1   TRANSACTIONAL VERSUS TRANSFORMATIONAL LEADERSHIP TRAITS (ADAPTED FROM NORTHOUSE[3])

Leadership Research: Transactional Versus Transformational

Transactional	Transformational
▪ Transaction (or exchange) of something the leader has that the follower wants	▪ Inspires followers to see beyond their self-interest
▪ Specifies roles and tasks	▪ Adapts to the needs and motives of followers
▪ Reward & punishment used as motivation	▪ Behaves in a way that engenders great trust
▪ "One-size-fits-all"	▪ The leader often relies on charisma

"What needs to happen for you to build great hospitals?" he asked, and they responded with a litany of complaints about government, insurers, and patients. He advised them to move beyond simply dealing with their problems if they wanted to achieve greatness.

Fair enough, but the constraints on hospitals are, in fact, very considerable, and increasing. There's no question that they have a negative effect on leaders' attitudes and behaviors toward proposed quality improvement initiatives.

Consolidation is roiling the profession. Mergers are creating ever more giant medical centers that threaten the existence of independent hospitals. Mergers among insurers have drained away much of hospitals' bargaining power. Hospitals' growing employment of physicians has substantially increased costs, often without matching increases in productivity. At the same time, the shortage of doctors is expected to reach 63,000 by 2015 according to the Association of American Medical Colleges.[4] The move toward electronic medical records continues to impose major financial burdens on hospitals and heavier workloads on healthcare workers. Government funding has dropped along with Medicare reimbursement. And the list goes on . . .

In our research, we came upon hospital leaders who threw up their hands when "the system" put a roadblock in the way of progress. The chief quality officer at a major academically affiliated hospital told us that a quality improvement effort had been shot down by the clinical executive board with the comment, "Oh, no, we can't ask our residents to date and time their orders." He blamed the decision on the board's inclination to favor academic priorities, such as writing papers and grants, and teaching, over clinical needs, and he dropped his proposal. At another site, the intensive care unit (ICU) director wanted to use a novel approach to reduce CLABSI in his unit because of an elevated infection rate and was stymied by the infection prevention staff. He had failed to further pursue the matter, so we asked why he didn't appeal the decision to someone in leadership. "You know," he said, "management changes so often. . . so that you kind of say, 'Well, is it worth working with them?' because if when you are done, you are just going to be starting all over again."

But effective leaders, we found, wherever they are in a hospital's hierarchy, don't take no for an answer. They find ways to accomplish their goals. The best C-suite leaders, for example, don't allow system challenges to keep them from their core mission—the cultivation of a culture of patient-centered clinical excellence.

There are innumerable definitions of leadership. Napoleon offered, "A leader is a dealer in hope." Lao Tzu, the ancient Chinese philosopher, said of the good leader: "when his work is done, his aim fulfilled, they will all say, 'We did this ourselves.'" We favor the straightforward definition of Peter G. Northouse, a preeminent scholar in leadership studies, from his book, *Leadership: Theory and Practice:* "Leadership is a process whereby an individual influences a group of individuals to achieve a common goal."[3] (See Box 5.2.)

Northouse described an invaluable distinction between two types of leadership. He called one "assigned leadership" because it is based on the position a person occupies in an organization. The other type he called "emergent leadership" because it emerges from an influential person in a group no matter what that person's position in the organization. In other words, you don't automatically become a leader because you're a manager. Warren Bennis and Burt Nanus put it succinctly in their book, *Leaders: Strategies for Taking Charge:* "Managers are people who do things right and leaders are people who do the right thing."

Box 5.2 KEY LEADERSHIP TRAITS (ADAPTED FROM NORTHOUSE[3])

Key Leadership Traits

Persistence
Intelligence
Integrity
Self-confidence
Sociability

THE ROLE OF HOSPITAL LEADERS

Hospital administrators and clinical chiefs can and should take on personal leadership roles in quality improvement initiatives. By simply mentioning a new infection prevention project as a reflection of the hospital's mission in their meetings and other encounters with staff members, they can help build powerful support for the project throughout the institution. They can stop by and listen in to a reporting session on the initiative, boosting the team's sense of purpose. They can include updates on the project's progress in their hospital-wide newsletter and online communications. They can make the degree of a person's support of quality initiatives a regular element of employee performance reviews. And top supervisors can provide backing when those leading an initiative run up against immovable roadblocks. "We kind of have an open door to senior management if we need to," an infection preventionist told us, describing an initiative. "I mean, I can go up and talk to the chief of staff or the medical director or CEO of the hospital if I needed to."

The familiar and much-praised "management by walking around" leadership approach is effective if the leader is looking and listening and communicating his vision for the hospital. But too many leaders view management by walking around as an exercise in nitpicking, a chance to show how all-seeing and important they are. We encountered a chief of staff like that: He would spot a minor problem, insist that it be corrected instantly, and wait around for the correction, forcing staff members to ignore more pressing matters. In one case, the problem was a dirty corner, and he had everyone trying to reach the janitor to come clean it up.

Leaders do have to be hardnosed, to hold their people accountable for results, but they need to pick their spots more carefully than that chief of staff. Though most problems yield to reason and compromise, some require a firm stand. Witness the familiar unwillingness of some physicians to fill out complete and timely medical records. Many hospitals allow their physicians to bend the rules, afraid of antagonizing those who help to keep the beds full. Yet when hospitals get tough with, say, a leading surgeon to the point of suspending him for a week or two, the result is often beneficial: The surgeon returns ready to abide by the medical records policy, and his surgical colleagues follow suit.

The chief of staff at an academically affiliated hospital gave us an example of her preference for dealing with problems head on, rather than letting them slide. One of her department heads received what she described as an "embarrassingly" poor audit score. She sat him down, read him the riot act, instructed him to improve his ways quickly—and sent a letter describing the situation to his university supervisor. The problem was soon resolved.

When there's staff turnover in a department, the boss faces mounting pressure to hire replacements rapidly because the remaining staff members are forced to take on extra duties. An infection preventionist leader we interviewed refused to fill a vacancy for a year because he wouldn't settle for second best. He was a strong advocate of the "hire hard, manage easy" school of leadership. After finding the right person, he said, "my life is so much better." As Donald Rumsfeld put it, "A's hire A's while B's hire C's."

PINPOINTING KEY LEADERSHIP BEHAVIORS

Some years ago, we studied 14 hospitals to see if we could identify the major characteristics of those leaders who were successful in implementing infection prevention practices.[5] We conducted 38 in-depth telephone interviews followed by 48 on-site interviews at 6 of the hospitals. The telephone interviews were with infection preventionists, hospital epidemiologists, infectious diseases physicians, and critical care nurse managers. The on-site interviews were primarily spread among the same group plus chiefs and directors, chairs and vice-chairs of medicine, and quality managers or medical directors of quality. These were the characteristics that stood out among those who led successful infection prevention projects, and they were confirmed in our more recent site visits and interviews (in total we have studied 46 hospitals and conducted more than 450 interviews):

- They were dedicated to establishing or maintaining a culture of clinical excellence—and were successful at communicating that patient-centered vision to their staff. When physicians and nurses live by a culture that puts patient safety first, they are inevitably more open to infection prevention initiatives. At one of the hospitals we studied, when staff members came to the CEO with a disagreement, she would routinely ask, "What's the best thing for the patient?" That would settle the matter. And we saw indications that her philosophy had been absorbed by her staff.

- They were solution-oriented, ready and able to overcome any and all barriers to success. Unlike those leaders quoted earlier, who blamed the system for their inaction, effective leaders found answers. A hospital epidemiologist reported that his hospital had been getting nowhere with a CAUTI prevention project because of a lack of nursing leadership. Finally, he teamed up with nurse managers and nurses to conduct a successful initiative to reduce the use of Foleys. "We partnered with managers instead of nursing leaders," he said.

- They were inspirational, not only in articulating their vision, but also in leading other staff members to take on leadership roles. We encountered an outstanding example in the person of a hospital epidemiologist at a private hospital. "We're inspired having somebody like him," said the lead infection preventionist. "He's got that mindset. It's all about the safety of the patient . . . not getting caught up so much on the politics and bureaucracy of it, just saying, 'O.K., let's make this work.' That in itself energizes us."

- They were careful strategists, preparing the ground for a project, ready to do the preliminary politicking and to use their personal prestige to pave the way for acceptance. As a chief of medicine told us, "I think most hospitals. . . have too many committees and are less productive in terms of what they accomplish. If I'm going to take a serious vote at. . . a committee, I want to know the vote's results before they're taken." In another hospital, an infection preventionist, faced with an administrator who had turned down the purchase of large drapes for central line insertions, began by getting his proposal approved by the infection control committee and then built support among physicians. "They drive the bus," he said, "so that's why we partner with doctors all the time." When he went back to the administrator, he said, he was able to prove that he had examined other options, that he had the backing of the physicians who would use the equipment, and that the coverings were supported in the literature—and he got his drapes.

For leaders at any level within a hospital to bring about a successful quality improvement intervention, creating a new behavioral norm requires all those legislative skills that Jim Collins spoke of, and that includes a goodly helping of emotional intelligence.

Emotional intelligence—it became known as EQ, or emotional quotient, by analogy with IQ, for intelligence quotient—first came to public attention in an article by two psychologists, John Mayer and Peter Salovey, in 1990.[6] They defined it as the "ability to monitor one's own and others' feelings and emotions, to discriminate among them, and to use this information to guide one's thinking and action." The authors brought together a number of scientific discoveries of the time, some of them dealing with how the brain regulates emotions.

A leader's emotional intelligence is not a matter of her being naturally friendly and sympathetic to other people. Nor is it simply a knack for sensing what other people are feeling, though that's a part of it. EQ requires some degree of thinking about feelings, your own and those of others, and consciously using those emotions to help make decisions and solve problems. It calls for you to develop rules about emotions that can guide your behavior—anger often yields to shame, for example. And it encompasses the ability to manage emotions, your own and those of others, to achieve your goals. If you know that a colleague who has expressed his anger toward you is likely to be feeling somewhat ashamed of himself the next day, you know that he may welcome a chance to make up and reconsider his position.

Thousands of schools around the world now teach EQ skills to students, and thousands of companies now apply emotional intelligence in judging whether to hire and promote employees and in training them to improve job performance. There is a Consortium for Research on Emotional Intelligence in Organizations that aids companies, such as American Express and Johnson & Johnson, and government agencies, such as the Defense Finance Accounting Service, by improving their use of EQ.

THE FOLLOWERS' RESPONSIBILITY

A well-developed emotional intelligence can help leaders in so many ways, but all the various attributes of the successful hospital leader that we have discussed point to one essential goal: By definition, any leader must have followers. But until Robert E. Kelley came along with his *Harvard Business Review* article, "In Praise of Followers," in 1988, nobody had bothered to give followers anything like the academic research accorded leaders—even though it's the followers who actually get the job done.

His first book[7] on the subject, *The Power of Followership*, in 1992, was a bestseller. When he began his work on followership, he wrote, "I felt like the odd person out. Executives, academics, and even people sitting next to me on airplanes questioned why I would bother with followership when leadership spurred the media attention, research funding, and high-paying corporate gigs. . . . At some point, I finally decided to put a stake in the ground. . . . "

Kelley identified five key types of followers:

- Alienated. They are mavericks who may be capable, but they tend to be highly cynical, and they have a healthy skepticism toward the organization.
- Conformists. They are the organization's "yes people," but they generally exercise limited independent thinking.

- Passivists. They lack initiative and any sense of responsibility. They require disproportionate supervision relative to their contribution.
- Pragmatists. They hug the middle of the road. They will do a good job but won't stick their necks out.
- Exemplary followers. They manage themselves and their work well, constantly improving their skills. They have a commitment to the organization and its vision. They are innovative and independent, willing to question their leaders.

As you may have noted, that description of exemplary followers bears a strong resemblance to our earlier description of successful leaders. As Kelley wrote, "Instead of seeing the leadership role as superior to and more active than the role of the follower, we can think of them as equal but different activities." Other researchers went on to claim that followership was itself a form of leadership, a skill set that could be and should be taught as a leadership requirement.[7]

Leaders should sit down with each of their immediate followers and explain the mission and vision of the organization. They need to describe what the follower's role is and how that role contributes to the mission. By the time the meeting is over, the follower should understand the standards by which his or her performance will be measured. And for their followers to achieve their full potential, leaders should schedule regular individual catch-up sessions, every month or so. That's how followers can be helped to become exemplary followers.

In the hospital setting, of course, some of the attributes of good followership are already in place. Most staff members in any hospital share a commitment to the institution and to the hospital's patient-centered vision. (Consider the clinical pharmacist who was monitoring adherence to the sedation and weaning protocols during an initiative to prevent ventilator-associated pneumonia at a hospital we studied. Unasked, he added head-of-bed elevation to the list of items he was checking. That's good followership.) As for being independent and willing to question leaders, that comes naturally to physicians and to at least some nurses.

THE POWER OF THE GROUP

When a hospital's leaders initiate a quality improvement intervention, however, they confront a daunting challenge. They must convince enough followers to alter their habitual way of proceeding to tip the balance of the institution toward a new set of habits. One of the greatest stumbling blocks in that process is the emotional weight of old habits—the old norm. Just because a leader asks them, followers don't willingly give up their norm. They are more likely to change their ways, though, if a new process gains a certain level of group approval.

That phenomenon is bred in our bones. Recent animal research has demonstrated the power of group norms. In a study of wild vervet monkeys,[8] for example, four groups were each presented with adjacent trays, blue-dyed corn in one, pink-dyed corn in the other. The colors were carefully chosen to attract the attention of both sexes—they represent the colors of the vervet's testicles. In two of the groups, the blue was more bitter-tasting than the pink, and vice versa for the other two groups. The members of all four groups opted for the more tasteful corn, regardless of its color, creating group preferences. Four months later, after a new cohort of infants matured enough for solid foods, the trays were put back in place, but this time neither the blue nor the pink corn was bitter-tasting. The infants overwhelmingly partook of the corn color their mothers ate. But when 10 adult male members of the four groups migrated to settle in new groups, they found that their new group favored corn of a different color from their original choice— and they switched to the local color, even though their association with that color had been negative. The power of the group norm outweighed their personal norm.

Yet it is specifically a group norm—the traditional attitudes and procedures for dealing with Foleys, central venous catheters, and mechanical ventilators—that the quality initiatives discussed in this book must overcome. The outstanding scholar of how that can happen, of how innovation spreads, is Everett M. Rogers, who was born on his family's farm in Iowa in 1931 and grew up expecting to follow in his father's footsteps. A visit to

Iowa State University changed his mind, and he eventually earned a PhD there in sociology and statistics.

In 1962, Rogers published *Diffusion of Innovations*. It describes the process whereby a new idea is accepted by a group or social system, starting with the innovators, who represent just 2.5% of the group. The idea begins to get a foothold with the early adopters (13.5%). It speeds up as it captures the early majority (about a third), and triumphs with the late majority (again, about a third). All that's left, then, is to wrap up the laggards (16%).[9]

Sometimes, the laggards take some convincing. When Rogers was a child, his father decided not to plant the then-new hybrid seed corn, which was said to be drought-resistant and had been adopted by a neighboring farmer. When a devastating drought struck Iowa that year, the Rogers corn wilted while the neighbor's crop flourished. The next year, Rogers Senior planted the hybrid.

The diffusion of an idea or innovation, Rogers said, "is essentially a process occurring through interpersonal networks." He tracked an individual's reactions to an idea or innovation through various stages, from her first exposure to the idea, to her active interest in learning more about it, to her deciding to try it to determine how useful or desirable it is, to her final adoption. All sorts of influences can affect that process, from political rallies to TV ads, but the reactions and experiences of the members of the individual's group are key.

When we have to make a decision, we listen to the advice of our families and friends and neighbors, the people we trust. If they buy a particular brand of refrigerator or car, if they are signing on to a new medical plan, we're inclined to follow suit. It just makes sense that people who are like us will be good guides. Their reactions to ideas and innovations are going to be similar to what ours would be since, after all, that's part of what makes us all members of the same group, the same social system. And in any event, it's just more comfortable to be doing what the majority of our group's members do.

No, we're not in the same class as the vervet monkeys, certainly not in the same genetics class—but the general principle holds. Though leaders can lean us in one or another direction, we tend to go along with the group consensus when confronted by an innovation. We trust the group.

In most cases, the arrival of an innovation, like a quality improvement initiative, forces us to contemplate changing the way we live in some way, large or small. Often, our reaction is annoyance. We don't want to be bothered; we're doing very nicely without the new device or idea.

So, Rogers asked, if you want to convince a group of people, many of them resistant, to accept a new idea or initiative, what's the most productive approach? His answer: Find members of the group who are generally admired and trusted and who believe in the new idea or initiative—and set them loose on the group as a whole. They are by far the best leaders for any kind of change. "Example is not the main thing in influencing others," Albert Schweitzer said, "it is the only thing."

And that is why most infection prevention initiatives today, like those we describe at the model hospital, rely so heavily on person-to-person contacts between members of a project team and the hospital staff. A physician champion is the natural person to convince other physicians to alter their attitudes toward the Foley, for example. A nurse champion is the natural person to convince other nurses that Foleys cause infection and should be removed with alacrity. Yes, the champions must be chosen with care. If the physician champion selected is unpopular with his colleagues or unknown to most of them, he is unlikely to get the job done. If the nurse champion lacks a warm and friendly personality, she is unlikely to inspire her colleagues to change their ways. But these caveats aside, the evidence of hundreds of initiatives supports the Rogers premise as the most efficient approach to revising a hospital's clinical norms.

That said, the hospital leadership still has an important responsibility in any initiative. As suggested earlier, the administrative and clinical leaders need to be supportive of the project, using their bully pulpit within the organization. Our studies do suggest that, although the administrative side may be very helpful, the major leadership burden falls on the clinical leaders, both nursing and physician leadership. If they are not engaged in visibly supporting an initiative, if they are not responsive to appeals from project leaders, if they are not respected within the hospital community, quality initiatives often flounder.

We have also found that hospitals whose leaders, administrative as well as clinical, have created or maintained a culture of excellence are likely to have successful quality initiatives. That's because such hospitals allow project champions to grow and flourish and because the sites accept such initiatives as opportunities for improvement.

At the hospital mentioned earlier, where the pharmacist took on an extra monitoring task, we learned how a variety of leaders can bring a quality improvement initiative to fruition. The initial impetus for the project came from the chief operating officer, who announced that the hospital was going to adopt standards from the highly regarded Institute for Healthcare Improvement (a nonprofit organization founded by Donald Berwick that has championed patient safety initiatives throughout the world). That inspired nursing leadership to consider ventilator-associated pneumonia prevention. The Critical Care Nurse Practice Committee picked up the leadership ball, reviewing the literature, and deciding that the chief point of attack would be bed elevation—making sure that the head of the bed of patients on a ventilator was at an elevation of at least 30 degrees to reduce the chance of aspiration.

A critical care nurse manager was a leader on the floor, organizing in-services, putting up educational posters, and talking up the initiative with colleagues. At the same time, this nurse champion monitored beds herself for six months. The hospital's overworked infection control staff was supportive but not actively involved in the project, though they were enthusiastic observers—"jumping up and down" about it, a nurse reported. Top-level management was not involved either. The project leaders were a nurse manager and a handful of other nurses, and when the initiative led to a drastic reduction in the incidence of pneumonia among patients on ventilators, it was the nurse managers and the bedside nurses on the floor who deserved the credit.

In the next chapter, we look at the problems encountered during the implementation of a quality improvement intervention, including a rogues' gallery of the three kinds of staff members who are responsible for most of those problems: active resisters, organizational constipators, and timeservers. We offer suggestions for coping with each of them.

SUGGESTIONS FOR FURTHER READING

Blackshear, P. B. (2004). The followership continuum: A model for increasing organizational productivity. *The Innovation Journal: The Public Sector Innovation Journal*, 9(1), 1–16.

In this paper, the author presents stages of followership within a model for measuring workforce performance level that he refers to as the Followership Continuum. The author proposes that, by focusing on assessing and developing the highest followership stages of the continuum, workforce productivity can be greatly improved.

Blanchard, K. H., & Johnson, S. (2003). *The one minute manager* (3rd ed.). New York, NY: William Morrow.

One of the most widely read management books, *The One Minute Manager* tells the story of a young man on a quest to "find out what really [makes] an effective manager tick." Through this concise, easy-to-read story, advice is shared in the form of three extremely practical "secrets": one minute goals; one minute praisings; and one minute reprimands.

Kelley, R. E. (1988, November-December). In praise of followers. *Harvard Business Review*, 66(6), 142–148.

In this article, the author argues that organizations stand or fall not only because of how well their leaders lead, but also how well their followers follow. Although many management books explore the traits necessary to be a strong leader, Kelley explores those necessary to encourage effective following.

Kotter, J. P. (1990). What leaders really do. *Harvard Business Review*, 68(3), 103–111.

In this classic paper that rings as true today as it did when it was first published over 20 years ago, Kotter argues that it is imperative for companies to realize that leadership is different from management. He goes on to dispute the idea that one is better than the other, and to show why they are both necessary for success in the business world.

Northouse, P. (2013). *Leadership: Theory and practice* (6th ed.). Thousand Oaks, CA: SAGE.

Used as the standard textbook at colleges and universities worldwide, this book is an accessible presentation of the major theories and models of leadership. The author has included practical exercises and case studies throughout. A must-have for anyone interested in the topic.

Saint, S., Kowalski, C. P., Banaszak-Holl, J., Forman, J., Damschroder, L., & Krein, S. L. (2010). The importance of leadership in preventing healthcare-associated infection: Results of a multisite qualitative study. *Infection Control and Hospital Epidemiology, 31*(9), 901–907.

In this article, Saint and colleagues follow up on preliminary data that indicated that hospital leadership played an important role in whether a hospital was engaged in infection prevention activities. They found that successful leaders (a) cultivated a culture of clinical excellence and effectively communicated it to staff; (b) focused on overcoming barriers and dealt directly with resistant staff or process issues that impeded prevention of healthcare-associated infection; (c) inspired their employees; and (d) thought strategically while acting locally, which involved politicking before crucial committee votes, leveraging personal prestige to move initiatives forward, and forming partnerships across disciplines.

Common Problems, Realistic Solutions

First they ignore you. Then they laugh at you. Then they fight you. And then . . . you win.

—MOHANDAS K. GANDHI

The nurse manager was an enthusiastic supporter of the bladder bundle, but her plans were opposed by the hospital's nurse executive. "She's a very energetic person and loves to try new things," the nurse executive said. "She doesn't realize it's not her kitchen so she can't make a new cake every day." In this case, the ill-fated "cake" happened to be the prevention initiative focused on catheter-associated urinary tract infection (CAUTI).

There are two basic kinds of problems to be resolved in undertaking a project to prevent healthcare-associated infections. Some barriers are of a practical, technical nature, the natural consequence of disrupting a system as complex as a hospital—new physicians' orders must be developed, bedside carts must be reconfigured. Other barriers are more personal in nature—the resistance of physicians, nurses, and administrators to a change they don't like because it's seen as mistaken or inconvenient or, as in the case of that nurse executive, because she sees it as challenging her authority and the status quo. In this chapter, we explore both kinds of problems, and offer some best-practice ideas for coping with them.

Our focus has shifted, though, from a single unit of our model, 250-bed hospital to the institution as a whole. With the success of the bladder bundle on 4 West, the administration has decided to go global. The elements of the bundle and the implementation approach will remain the same, including the daily catheter patrol, for example. But the major expansion of the intervention generates substantial new challenges.

One of the reasons 4 West was chosen to pilot the intervention was the positive attitude its leaders and bedside nurses had exhibited toward earlier improvement efforts. Now, the project leaders will have to cope with the full gamut of staff reactions, the total range of emotional responses in more than a dozen different units and departments. At the same time, the demands on various parts of the hospital will increase: the supply department will start receiving multiple requests for condom catheters or bladder scanners; the infection prevention department will have to organize and analyze copious new reams of data.

The intervention will also require a somewhat new leadership structure, though no such change might be needed in a smaller facility. Our executive sponsor will stay on, as will the project manager, a major advantage since the lessons the manager learned and the contacts she made dealing with 4 West will be a substantial help in coordinating the hospital-wide rollout. The nurse and physician champions are taking on new roles in the intervention as the go-to people for their counterparts throughout the hospital: there will be a nurse champion for each unit on the medical floor as well as a nurse and physician champion for the emergency department and for each intensive care unit (ICU). In that way, the project leaders hope to be able to tailor the intervention to the particularities of the various units. One unit, for example, might have an unusually large percentage of patients who are incontinent, leading the team to arrange for extra nursing assistance.

Any quality improvement enterprise can encounter a variety of baked-in challenges. The big teaching hospitals are slow-moving and bureaucratic with a tendency to consider themselves special, as in, "our floor patients are so sick they'd be in the ICU at any other hospital." Their tenured faculty members are often less interested in clinical matters, such as quality initiatives, than they are in research, the primary track for promotion.

- Clinical staffs everywhere are already strained by cutbacks in personnel and physical resources. So an emergency department might rule out the use of intermittent straight catheters as Foley alternatives because of the extra nursing time required.
- Existing organizational policies can conflict with the recommendations of the intervention. An obstetrics department order, for instance, may call for the automatic placement of an indwelling catheter for every patient receiving epidural analgesia.
- Rigid employment rules make it difficult to remove uncooperative or underperforming personnel. As one infection preventionist sarcastically put it: "You don't get fired if you work for this outfit; well, maybe if you kill four people and they find three of the bodies."
- Each project has to compete with other quality initiatives for staff time and resources, and the initiatives are proliferating.
- Some physicians are going to resist any kind of new technology including the electronic patient records system.

Given these and additional barriers, we have provided a list of common barriers and possible solutions that hospitals have found successful. (See Table 6.1.)

Staff misunderstandings can be a major obstacle to a successful quality improvement intervention. For instance, the bladder bundle accepts the use of an indwelling catheter for prolonged immobilization, say for a patient with a lumbar spine fracture. We encountered nurses who interpreted that to mean that they should use a Foley for patients on bed rest. Some hospitals found that using the condom catheter instead of the Foley was problematic since the condom catheter chosen rarely stayed on the male patient. The constant leakage of urine on the patient's bedsheets and

TABLE 6.1   BARRIERS AND SOLUTIONS

BARRIERS TO SUCCESSFUL INTERVENTION	POSSIBLE SOLUTIONS
Some nurses may not be on board with indwelling urinary catheter removal	▪ Get buy-in before implementation. For example, ask, "Whom do we have to convince on this floor?" Have that person help to develop the plan or participate in the education for that unit. ▪ Listen to nurses' concerns and address them to nurses' satisfaction.

Lack of or problems with nurse champions	▪ Identify the types of champions who work in your organization. Do not use a one-size-fits-all strategy. For example:
	  ▫ Use nurse educators as champions.
	  ▫ Have more than one nurse champion (i.e., co-champions).
	▪ Recognize nurse champions via such mechanisms as certificates of recognition, annual evaluation appraisals, newsletters, and notifying the nursing director.

Lack of physician buy-in of new practice and/ or physicians are resistant to change in general	▪ Provide data to physicians about urinary catheter use, monthly indwelling urinary catheter prevalence, and CAUTI rates.
	▪ Provide one-on-one education (evidence-based and safety oriented).
	▪ Engage medical leadership support, for example, the chief of staff.
	▪ Involve physicians as much as possible in planning, education, and implementation; include physicians on your team.
	▪ Identify a physician champion who will:
	  ▫ Meet with other physicians to get them on board.
	  ▫ Back up nurses when there's a disagreement.
	  ▫ Present evidence such as highlighting how often physicians who have patients with indwelling urinary catheters forget about them.

(continued)

TABLE 6.1 (Continued)

BARRIERS TO SUCCESSFUL INTERVENTION	POSSIBLE SOLUTIONS
Lack of physician champion	■ In institutions where there are good nurse-physician working relationships, most physicians may be willing to go along with recommendations by nurses, especially if the new practice is viewed as a "nursing initiative." ■ Also see previous discussion about overcoming resistant physicians.
Leadership does not see CAUTI as a priority	■ Prepare and present a business case to help convince leadership that the time and cost factors for implementing the new practice will be worth it. ■ Be sure leadership receives monthly CAUTI rates and catheter use data.
General guidance	■ Get people on the team who feel CAUTI is worth addressing. ■ Highlight staff who have adopted the new practice. ■ Know the system and how to get practice changes through relevant committees.
Nurses schedules are inflexible, so difficult to do education	■ Rather than having the nurses attend education sessions, bring the education to the bedside. Do competencies on the unit, talking with nurses one-to-one during the point prevalence assessments. ■ Incorporate education on CAUTI into annual competency testing.
Nurses are not confident speaking with physicians about removal	■ Find a physician champion to support nurse requests for removal. ■ Have the nurse manager prompt nurses to speak with physicians. ■ Provide education on communication.

(continued)

TABLE 6.1 (Continued)

BARRIERS TO SUCCESSFUL INTERVENTION	POSSIBLE SOLUTIONS
Resistance to early indwelling urinary catheter removal from surgeons and urologists	▪ Have the physician champion present at a medical staff meeting about indications and nonindications for indwelling urinary catheters. ▪ Work with the physician assistants to discontinue indwelling urinary catheters within 1 or 2 days after surgery. ▪ Engage a surgeon and/or urologist as a physician champion and work with that person to establish conditions under which the catheter can be removed.

gown—caused by a substandard product or improper placement technique—led to unhappy patients and unhappy nurses.

Efforts to reduce infection rates can also be sabotaged by the inadequate training or proficiency of those who are placing the Foleys and straight catheters. One nurse executive had occasion to evaluate competencies of a group of nurses' aides: "I had a mannequin down there, and what I saw was kind of scary." Nurses' aides trained by registered nurses (RNs) would, in turn, train new aides, and errors would compound. In that hospital, aides and RNs now refresh their catheter insertion skills annually, using real people as well as mannequins.

In addition to monitoring the reactions of the staff to a quality initiative, the project leaders need to keep a wary eye on their own team. A nurse champion with a patronizing attitude toward bedside nurses can undermine the most carefully planned project. And beware the team member who always explains away unexpected personnel problems as the result of staff resistance, a scapegoating technique to divert attention from his or her own mistakes. It's important for the team as a whole to remember that resistance, for all its annoyance, can sometimes be extremely valuable, signaling a weakness in the project that requires correction—or a special circumstance that demands an exception to the recommendations of the bladder bundle.

Leaders of change efforts of any kind need to keep in mind the power of positive deviance, an approach to problem-solving that looks for those outliers in every community whose tendency to avoid status quo thinking and behavior can reveal important new solutions for the community as a whole.[1] The positive deviance approach was first applied in the 1990s in Vietnam villages where the majority of children suffered from malnutrition. A handful of outlier families with well-nourished children were studied. They were found to be feeding their children foods that the other families viewed as inappropriate for children, including shrimp and sweet potato greens. Once the community was convinced to try that diet, the malnutrition faded.

One hospital with an eye for outliers creates a special committee when it is about to scale up an intervention. The committee consists of physicians and nurses with a reputation for criticizing such projects. At meetings, the committee members are urged to report what they see as problems in the proposed intervention, and the project leaders take careful notes. Along with the expected knee-jerk complaints, the leaders generally uncover some real shortcomings. As an added benefit, the fault-finding members of the committee, having vented their views, tend to maintain a neutral position toward the intervention once it is underway.[2]

The most important single factor in any such project, of course, is the quality of the individual hospital's culture. It's a word that has been greatly devalued, its meaning stretched beyond recognition, but to paraphrase Justice Potter Stewart's famous comment about pornography, we know a dysfunctional culture when we see it. The staff members are territorial rather than supportive; averse to change rather than invested in their unit's efficiency; obedient rather than empowered. Quality interventions are unlikely to flourish in such arid soil.

In the day-to-day operation of a quality improvement project, the leaders' greatest challenge is to convince the clinical staff to adopt new goals and practices. In our view, there are three types of staff members who present the most problems for an initiative: Active resisters openly oppose the intervention; organizational constipators get in the way; and timeservers undermine it by reason of their very laziness and indifference. We discuss them next in that same sequence, in emotionally descending order: The timeservers are the most difficult to convert into project supporters.

ACTIVE RESISTERS

Physicians and nurses among the active resisters often cite common reasons for their attitude, including a shared distaste for any project that rocks the boat, as in, "If it ain't broke, don't fix it." However, the underlying reasons for their opposition, the ways in which it manifests, and the best responses to their behavior are often different, enough so that we believe the two groups warrant separate treatment.[3]

The most extreme emergence of the resistant physician takes place during an encounter between a physician and a nurse during rounds outside a patient's room, by a patient's bed, or on a telephone. The nurse says something like, "Dr. Jones, according to the bladder bundle, I think the Foley should be removed," and Dr. Jones replies, "After you go to medical school, Miss Smith, you can tell me what to do." More than one staff member has told us that story, and others have the physician saying, "You are just a nurse. Don't question me," or, "Who asked you?"

That sounds as though the physicians' motivations had more to do with their ego than anything else—their judgment had been challenged—and certainly ego plays a role. Physicians have traditionally been trained to see themselves as independent and self-regulating, the ultimate authority charged with life-saving responsibility. They do not expect to be monitored or corrected in their medical practice, and certainly not by a non-physician in front of other hospital personnel.

Yet there can be a variety of other reasons behind their resistance to a quality initiative. In some cases, a different kind of embarrassment may be at play, because the physicians simply did not know that their patient even had a Foley or had forgotten it was there. One study[4] found that attending physicians were unaware that their patient had an indwelling catheter 38% of the time, and the inappropriate catheters were more often missed than the appropriate ones. Many inappropriate Foleys remain in place until there is some complication related to the catheters or until just before the patients are discharged.

Physicians in general, and surgeons in particular, sometimes oppose an intervention because of a tendency to be paranoid by profession. Any kind of change, they fear, will throw them off their game and threaten the modus operandi they have so carefully developed, with possibly dire consequences for both patient and physician. Resident physicians don't want to risk straying beyond what they've just been taught.

As suggested earlier, physicians may also resist quality improvement interventions because they are doubters: They have seen too many new theories disproven, too many "revolutionary" new techniques abandoned. Reports of fraud in scientific studies have become all too familiar. And they simply don't believe that all of the changes required by the intervention are scientifically valid or necessary. Indeed, as discussed in Chapter 3, some of the items in the bladder bundle are based more on common sense and observational studies than on rigorous randomized controlled trials. Physicians also have a tendency to view a quality initiative as research rather than as real medical practice. They see a research project as temporary, to be ignored until it disappears, while they get on with the serious work.

Underlying the opposition of some physicians—and nurses, as well—is their conviction that catheters and urinary tract infections represent an inferior order of medical problem. Why, they wonder, are we being pestered about such a minor matter when we are battling cancer, heart disease, and the like? A qualitative study found that a number of physicians interviewed simply did not believe that CAUTI posed a significant risk to their patients, particularly when compared to such infections as central line-associated bloodstream infection (CLABSI) and ventilator-associated pneumonia (VAP). As a result, CAUTI prevention was not a priority.[5]

At one institution, as the CAUTI intervention was starting, the hospital leadership decided that a urinary catheter reminder linked to a physician's order for a urinary catheter should be developed to engage doctors in the project. The staff member assigned that task first went to check out the institution's catheter policy in general—and discovered that there was none. Physicians who wanted Foleys placed gave verbal instructions to the nurses, and didn't even bother to write orders for the catheters.

Resistance by older physicians was especially problematic at one small, rural hospital. A director of quality described her institution as "the Rip Van Winkle of hospitals." The physicians, she said, have a "captain of the ship mentality." And when the "cash cow" surgeon refuses to abide by the bladder bundle, she added, "Do you think anybody is going to hold him accountable?"

In fact, hospitals have traditionally looked upon doctors as their customers—they who bring in the patients—but that has been changing. Many leading hospitals today are reshaping that relationship. They see patient care as more team-based than doctor-centered, with the nurse a full partner. They are demanding that physicians join them in treating the patient as the new customer-in-chief, and support the innovations that serve that customer's safety. Younger independent physicians and hospitalists are more likely to have heard and accepted that message than older practitioners.

At our model hospital, physicians who ignore bladder bundle practices because they doubt their scientific validity find themselves collared by the project's physician champion in the physicians' lounge or after a staff meeting. They are shown scientific studies describing the impressive drop in infections following bladder bundle interventions, especially after the timely removal of Foleys. They are shown statistics on the substantial incidence of CAUTI in their own hospital, including its financial impact. Finally, the physician champion acknowledges that there is always some element of risk in adopting a new policy, but he challenges the resister physician by asking, in effect, "How about the risk to your patients if you don't go along with the change?"

Each weekday of the first weeks of the hospital-wide intervention at the model hospital, the bedside nurses on catheter patrol indicate on the template and on the paper chart the status of their patients' Foleys including why they are in place. If an appropriate indication is not identified, they inform the physician that it is time to remove the Foley. Whether that is done in person or on a telephone, the intervention calls for that contact to be made each day an inappropriate Foley is present. And even for a habitual physician resister, that can have an effect. A bedside nurse told us, "The doctors catch on after a while. They get sick of listening to us, and they don't like phone calls."

Early in the intervention at the model hospital, as a way of easing doctors and nurses into the changes, a catheter reminder has been attached to the physician notes on patients' charts, on paper and in the electronic record. As noted previously, this low-cost system calls the physician's attention to the Foley and includes the basic components of the bladder bundle. Reminders can be effective, but one warning: It's so easy to add them to the computer system that there is danger of reminder overload. Hospitals need to develop ways to prioritize reminders in order to keep them under control.

After a week of reminders, when there is still some physician resistance, the model hospital posts a 48-hour default stop order for each Foley, indicating when it should be removed. The name of the hospital's medical director is prominently displayed on the order to further encourage cooperation. The stop order appears on patients' paper charts and on computerized patient records, and, when the date arrives, the template generates an electronic alert. In addition to the two kinds of reminders, some hospitals, faced with unco-operative doctors, have required physicians to sign plastic tape flags attached to the reminder sheets, indicating that they have been made aware of the bladder bundle requirements. Those who failed to do so were sent alphanumeric pages, a much more intrusive step, a forceful reminder of a reminder.

In many if not most hospitals, a doctor's order is required before a nurse is allowed to remove a Foley. As a result, when a nurse observes that a Foley should come out according to the bladder bundle standard, she must reach out to the physician until she finds him, even if it takes hours or days. We believe that is too long a time and too dangerous a policy. If there is any substantial delay, the nurse should be empowered to remove the catheter.

In its negotiations with resisting physicians, the project team at the model hospital treats them with respect and consideration and an appeal to their collegiality. Team members constantly remind each other that the majority of doctors and nurses, including the active resisters, have gone into healthcare to help people, certainly not to harm them. One project manager likes to recall an experiment in which three different signs were placed at a hospital's hand-washing stations over a two-week period.[6] One sign said that washing would keep the user from catching diseases, the second said washing would keep patients from catching diseases, and a third sign, serving as a control, had a generic message. Compared with the other signs, the patient-oriented sign inspired a 33% increase in the quantity of disinfectant and soap used at each station.

Eventually, with a handful of doctors still resisting the intervention, and expressing their opposition openly on rounds and at staff meetings, the model hospital's project team decides it needs topside help. The physician champion and project manager appeal to the hospital's medical director, and he agrees to send a stiff e-mail to each of the holdouts demanding their cooperation. If that fails, the hospital's administrative and clinical leaders have decided, they will give the offenders a stark choice: Cease their resistance or leave the hospital. If the patient is, in fact, the customer, they agree, the hospital cannot continue to tolerate physicians who will not put the patient's safety first.

Nurses become active resisters because they, like their physician counterparts, prefer the status quo, but their motivations are very different. Many of the resisters are veteran nurses who have spent their careers using the Foley both to lighten their workload and as a convenient tool for measuring urinary flow. They have, for example, used Foleys in patients who urinate frequently. As one nurse put it: "Some of the ladies go maybe 100 cc every 15 to 20 minutes, and you're in there constantly answering the lights." The resisters insist that the Foley alternatives, such as frequently toileting the ambulatory patients or using bedpans, take precious time away from other patients who may have greater need of their care. The impact of these longtime nurse resisters is compounded because they are the people to whom new and younger nurses go for advice.

For some nurse resisters, their main complaint centers on the need to alert physicians about the requirements of the bladder bundle for patients with Foleys. Some of these nurses insist that the decision to use or not use a Foley is the business of the physician, not the nurse's responsibility. Others find it impossible to challenge physicians under any circumstances.

There are other aspects of the intervention that stir nurses' opposition because they increase the workload. Collecting data on Foley use, for example, can be complicated and time consuming. In hospitals without an electronic database, paper records must be gone through. Sometimes catheterizations go undocumented, so the catheter patrol has to check under each patient's bed sheets. Determining whether a patient has a urinary tract infection can also be a lengthy process. A positive urine culture, for example, may or may not be definitive depending upon whether the patient meets a set of qualifying symptoms—symptoms that can vary depending upon the patient's age and ailments. If the patient is immuno-compromised, for instance, she may not spike a fever with an infection.

Supporting the nurses' opposition is their general belief that urinary tract infection is not a serious concern. "Let's think about it," an infection preventionist said. "The majority of our RNs are still female, and they've had hundreds of urinary tract infections in their lifetime. They did not die." In fact, they simply took narrow-spectrum antimicrobials, and the problem went away. We found that attitude to be all but universal in the hospitals we studied. When a patient falls, a clinical executive told us, he dispatches aides to get all the facts, to check procedures on every shift, to call meetings. "But if we get a Foley infection," he continued, "nobody says, 'Oooo, let's have a huddle and see how it happened.'"

The nurses' opposition to the project takes several forms. Sometimes they simply ignore the initiative, asking physicians to order a Foley regardless of whether it meets the bladder bundle appropriateness criteria or failing to speak to physicians about its timely removal. They may neglect to share information about patients with Foleys with their counterparts at shift change. They may also find ways to game the system.

The electronic medical records, for all their efficiency, provide opportunities for a workaround. Some hospitals use a scoring algorithm to help determine whether a catheter should be removed. Nurse resisters know what number is needed to make it appear that the catheter should stay in place, and use it rather than the number appropriate to the particular patient. In other hospitals, the electronic checklist of approved indications for ordering a catheter (or for keeping one in place) is followed by an "other" category. Resister nurses and doctors connive in checking that category when, in fact, there is no medical reason to place a Foley or to keep one in place.

We learned of one hospital that seemed to be doing well with a bladder bundle intervention on most counts, but then officials noticed that there was a strange surge in the number of cases of bladder outlet obstruction, at least as reflected in the reasons cited for maintaining a Foley on the medical records template. The officials concluded that the intervention might not be going as well as they thought.

At the model hospital, the project team has developed some specific solutions for individual problems posed by nurse resisters. It has eliminated the nurse-physician confrontation over removal of a Foley by empowering nurses to take out the catheter as called for by the bladder bundle without obtaining the physician's approval. In units with a larger-than-usual ratio of patients who urinate frequently, "small zones" have been established so that nurses who had been responsible for nine such patients were now responsible for seven. In other units where nurses have been feeling harried because of the intervention, nurses' aides are now instructed to devote more of their time to toileting patients. Hourly rounding has been instituted, which saves nurses time in the long run. (In our experience, when nurses say a patient needs to urinate every 15 minutes, it's generally an exaggeration—it just seems that short a time!)

The model hospital has also sought ways to make the right thing to do the easy thing to do, integrating each new quality improvement project with earlier safety initiatives. The hourly rounds for the bladder bundle intervention, for instance, were compatible with an intervention aimed at preventing falls. We learned of another hospital where a project on pressure ulcers accommodated the bladder bundle: The use of absorbent pads for the ulcer initiative served as a helpful alternative for catheter use for incontinence concerns.

To create a more positive culture around the intervention, a team effort, the hospital has posted the Foley prevalence rate and CAUTI rates on boards in all the units, showing nurses the results of their work. Those who are cooperating with the project are recognized with praise and assured that their good work will be included in annual staff evaluations. Staff meeting time is set aside to report on the progress and challenges of the initiative.

Nurse champions spend one-on-one time with resisters, often putting less emphasis on bringing down the hospital's CAUTI rates and more on the benefits of the bladder bundle for the nurses' patients—the discomfort and possible internal injury of the Foley versus the chance to get up and around and out of the hospital sooner. The appeal is to the nurse resister's dedication to her patients' welfare.

Before moving on to discuss organizational constipators and timeservers, we should mention another species of active resister—the patient and/or the patient's family. Patients who are worried about soiling themselves or who want to stay in bed will appeal to their physicians and nurses to maintain a Foley in place, even when it is not needed. And the device is so routine and of secondary concern for the clinical staff that they will often go along. "You know what," a physician told an infection preventionist, "they're laying there. They're miserable and they want the Foley. So let them have it." Families also sometimes request a Foley because they worry the patient will fall if he or she leaves the bed.

At the model hospital, nurses are trained to explain to patients about the potential damage and discomfort the catheters can cause, including a false feeling of the need to urinate. They emphasize the efficiency of Foley alternatives for the bedridden, and for those who are able, the importance of getting up and around to aid in recovery. Patients and families are also given a one-page explanation of these issues.

ORGANIZATIONAL CONSTIPATORS

Our use of the word *constipators* is somewhat tongue in cheek, but the term does clinically describe the impact these people—primarily mid- to high-level executives—can have on a quality improvement initiative.[3] And that impact can be considerable, even though the organizational constipators generally have no animus toward the particular works they are gumming up. They are, in effect, disinterested resisters of the initiative, and they come in two basic varieties.

Some of these people simply enjoy exercising their power. At one hospital, for example, the lead quality manager told us that after attending the first day of training for a project to reduce infections, she was forbidden to attend the second day by the chief nurse. No reason was given, and the chief nurse was not opposed to the project. The manager's explanation: It was a "control issue." The chief nurse viewed any independent action by an underling as an affront. Another such person might consider any effort to alter the status quo as a threat to his or her power. What distinguishes these kinds of organizational constipators is that their actions are purposeful.

Their counterparts exercise their power by failing to take action. Memos pile up in their inboxes and overload their e-mail accounts. A physician described his chief of staff: "Somebody who will nod their head and say, 'Well, let me think about it.'" He would keep bringing up an idea he had proposed, and the chief of staff wouldn't remember it, so the physician would have to go back into his own e-mail and resend an old message, adding, "Did you ever make a decision on this?" We heard stories of administrators who kept putting off the hiring of replacement nurses or signing off on purchase orders for lab equipment. An infection preven-tionist told of having a "huge problem" with an executive who "needs to do certain things and he just doesn't do them."

Aside from the direct damage that organizational constipators can do to safety initiatives, they can also lower staff morale and sour professional relationships, both of which are so essential to an initiative's success. The physician quoted earlier put it this way: "You just lose energy." A key prob-lem with organizational constipators is that their bosses think they are effective workers, whereas their underlings cannot believe the constipa-tors still have their jobs.

Organizational constipators are more difficult to cope with than active resisters, in part because their negative effect on a quality improvement intervention is a function of their normal operating style. There is no upset over extra work, no quarrel with the science of the bladder bundle, no negative attitude toward a particular nurse champion—attitudes of the active resister that at least lend themselves to being changed. In the case of the organizational constipator, the barrier to a successful intervention is rooted in some basic personality traits.

The managers of initiatives often try to work around these people. At one hospital, where the director of nursing was a notorious roadblock, the project manager told her little about the bladder bundle initiative and went over her head if there was a problem. A quality manager in a similar situation commented, "Basically, if I keep off the radar, I can do what I need." Some hospitals revise their organizational charts so that these troublemakers retain their title but their responsibilities are reassigned and they can do less damage.

A potentially more effective strategy was described by a hospital director: "Well, I think if you have a systematic way of addressing major issues through an executive board . . . Essentially we've brought a particular person who's known for . . . having strong opinions into these discussions and so we are able to vet them." The director explained the hazards of working around these individuals: "I think so often organizations take that person and keep them out because they're going to block maybe something that you wanted, and we put them over here instead of bringing them into the fold and . . . I've seen that in a couple of specific situations where it's been so helpful to have that person there and have the dialogue, and in a couple of instances, you know, they changed their mind or turned into a supporter of it."[3]

Eventually, though, some institutions run out of patience with organizational constipators. "The tough approach is what we've done here," a chief of medicine told us, "and that is, they're gone." Otherwise, hospitals can wait until such a person leaves or retires. When the opportunity does appear, they need to take their time in finding a replacement to make sure they're not simply trading one problem for another.

TIMESERVERS

"I don't have a clue what to do with either the stupid or the lazy," the chief of surgery said. "I have no way to make them work better." The people who fit the category we call "timeservers" are more likely to be lazy than stupid. They are essentially serving out their time, doing the least possible. Quality improvement initiatives are someone else's problem; they don't stick their necks out for anyone.

Even when a timeserver nurse has been fully briefed about, say, the bladder bundle, and the importance of removing a Foley in a timely manner, she'll find ways to do nothing. We learned of a nurse who promised her supervisor that she would talk with a doctor about removing a Foley over the weekend. When the supervisor returned on Monday, nothing had been done. Timeservers seldom follow through.

They take the course of least resistance: Do what the doctor says. If the patient wants to keep the Foley in place, don't bother discussing with her the pros and cons of that decision. In fact, keep a Foley in patients as long as possible because it's easier that way.

Short of having them fired, which is often a problem because of union rules, hospitals can try to change the behavior of timeservers by giving them daily reminders of the elements of a safety intervention and having an authority figure frequently reinforce the reminders.

We also favor another, admittedly demanding, approach for coping with timeservers as a group. We have observed that they tend to multiply in institutions burdened by a culture of mediocrity. If the leadership of a hospital is satisfied with second best, the environment will be ripe for timeserving. The cure is drastic: a conversion to a culture of excellence. It requires that the hospital instill a devotion to patient-centered, high-quality care in each and every unit, along with the full-bore support of quality improvement initiatives. Eventually, the psychological effect on timeservers would be comparable to what happens when a shopper finds herself in a Whole Foods store without a reusable bag. "She will run back to the car to get a reusable bag," a physician told us, "because people look at you funny in that store if you don't have one." If a unit or a floor of a hospital is dedicated to a patient-safety initiative, timeservers who don't shape up will be seen as shirkers and shunned. If that doesn't bring them around, nothing will. We provide, below, an overview of the three types of health-care workers who bedevil quality interventions along with a summary of some field-tested approaches to cope with them. (See Box 6.1.)

In the following chapter, the focus turns to the task of sustainability: How can a hospital hold onto the progress it has made during the course of a quality improvement intervention?

Box 6.1 **STYLES OF PERSONNEL BARRIERS (ADAPTED FROM SAINT ET AL.[3])**

CHALLENGING STAFF STYLES

1. Active resisters to a change in practice are pervasive, whether an attending physician, resident physician, or nurse. Successful efforts to overcome active resistance include the following:

   a. Data feedback comparing local infection rates to national rates.

   b. Data feedback comparing rates of compliance with the rates of others in the same area.

   c. Effective championing by an engaged and respected change agent who can speak the language of the staff he or she is guiding (e.g., a surgeon to motivate other surgeons).

   d. Participation in collaborative efforts that generally align hospital leadership and clinicians with the goal of reducing healthcare-associated infection.

2. Organizational constipators—mid- to high-level executives— act as insidious barriers to change in practice. Once leadership recognizes the problem and the negative effect on other staff, various techniques can be used to overcome these barriers.

   a. Include the organizational constipator early in group discussions in order to improve communication and obtain buy-in.

   b. Work around the individual, realizing that this is likely a shorter-term solution.

   c. Terminate the constipator's employment.

   d. Take advantage of turnover opportunities when the constipator leaves the organization by hiring a person who has a very high likelihood of being effective.

(Continued)

Box 6.1 (Continued)

3. Timeservers are essentially serving out their time, doing the least possible. These staff members are the hardest to overcome. Short of firing them, some suggestions include:
   a. Provide daily reminders of the elements of the safety intervention and have an authority figure frequently reinforce the reminders.
   b. Promote a culture of excellence.

SUGGESTIONS FOR FURTHER READING

Krein, S. L., Damschroder, L., Kowalski, C. P., Forman, J., Hofer, T. P., & Saint, S. (2010). The influence of organizational context on quality improvement and patient safety efforts in infection prevention: A multi-center qualitative study. *Social Science and Medicine*, 71(9), 1692–1701.
In this article, the authors closely examine quality improvement efforts and the implementation of recommended practices to prevent central line-associated bloodstream infection (CLABSI) in U.S. hospitals. They compare and contrast the experiences among hospitals to better understand how and why certain hospitals are more successful with practice implementation. Their findings provide important insights about how different quality improvement strategies might perform across organizations with differing characteristics.

Krein, S. L., Kowalski, C. P., Harrod, M., Forman, J., & Saint, S. (2013). Barriers to reducing urinary catheter use: A qualitative assessment of a statewide initiative. *JAMA Internal Medicine*, 173(10), 881–886.
Krein and colleagues purposefully sampled 12 hospitals that were participating in the Michigan Health and Hospital Association Keystone Center for Patient Safety statewide program to reduce unnecessary use of urinary catheters (the bladder bundle). The authors interviewed key informants to identify ways to enhance catheter-associated urinary tract infection prevention efforts based on the experiences of these hospitals. In the article, the authors present barriers to implementation and strategies to address them.

Saint, S., Kowalski, C. P., Banaszak-Holl, J., Forman, J., Damschroder, L., & Krein, S. L. (2009). How active resisters and organizational constipators affect health care-acquired infection prevention efforts. *Joint Commission Journal on Quality and Patient Safety*, 35(5), 239–246.
The authors collected qualitative data from phone and in-person interviews with hospital staff from a national study to determine the barriers to implementing

evidence-based practices to prevent healthcare-associated infection, with a specific focus on the role played by hospital personnel. They found that, in particular, two types of personnel—active resisters and organizational constipators—impeded infection prevention activities, and that, to overcome these barriers, hospital personnel used several approaches.

Toward Sustainability

We are what we repeatedly do. Excellence then, is not an act, but a habit.

—ARISTOTLE

"Nobody's going to sit back and be comfortable," the infection preventionist insisted. Her 500-bed suburban hospital had just completed a successful intervention to reduce its central line-associated bloodstream infection (CLABSI) rate, but she and her colleagues were not resting on their laurels. "You're going to push one another to go to that next level," she told us, "because having value and feeling like you make a difference is what makes you happy in your work."

In the quality improvement field, the ability to sustain and even improve a successful initiative is the Holy Grail, Ahab's white whale. Various managerial studies suggest that up to 70% of organizational change efforts simply don't survive. Once an initiative stops being an institutional focus, once an organization moves on to other projects, there's a natural tendency to revert to old ways. The damage may be substantial when a bank's change program lacks legs, but the demise of a hospital's quality improvement project—to reduce a healthcare-associated infection, for example—can have dire consequences for hundreds or thousands of patients.

For all the research about program sustainability, there is no valid, tested formula for doing it right. That's because the institutions involved are different from each other in so many ways, including their personnel, their policies, and their culture, not to mention the resources they are willing to commit to any given project. No single set of procedures fits them all. Yet there is a body of best practices that can help a hospital hold onto its quality improvement gains.

THE IMPORTANCE OF EARLY PLANNING

At our model hospital, the institution-wide intervention to prevent catheter-associated urinary tract infection (CAUTI) has run its 18-month course. Foley usage has been cut dramatically, leading to a sustained 30% to 35% CAUTI reduction throughout the hospital. A month before the intervention's end, the original leaders of the project team meet with the executive sponsor to review their work together and discuss what lies ahead: maintaining the progress to date. They know that hospitals too often jump from one change process to another without consolidating their advances. They know that even among institutions that recognize the importance of early planning for sustainability, too many give it lip service and nothing more.

In the model hospital, as noted earlier, sustainability was on the agenda from the start. The leaders of the initial intervention were carefully chosen with an eye to their staying power, and team members accepted their posts with the understanding that it would be an ongoing commitment. When the initiative scaled up, that same commitment was made by the new champions in the emergency department, the intensive care units, the operating rooms, and the individual floor units. The time requirements would be heaviest during the intervention phase, of course, but everyone knew that they would be needed after the formal initiative ended, as well. They also knew that their participation would continue to boost their annual staff evaluation.

At the prevention team's meeting, participants ask themselves how well the hospital is positioned to hold onto its CAUTI prevention gains. To what degree have the mandates of the bladder bundle become institutionalized?

Do the physicians and nurses automatically resist inserting Foleys that fail to meet appropriateness criteria? Do they remove Foleys when the catheters are no longer needed?

The team members happily agree that the basic elements of the bladder bundle have, in fact, become routine practice at the hospital. This will make their task much simpler. The director of acute care at a hospital described the sustainability of a CAUTI prevention initiative in her hospital in down-to-earth terms: "It's an everyday thing that we roll with."

Another advantage the team recognizes is their hospital's continuing culture of excellence. Just as it set the table for a successful CAUTI prevention intervention, the shared commitment to excellence underpins the sustainability of this and any such quality initiative.

THE PROJECT TEAM'S DUTIES

At the project team's meeting, the leaders agree that the lines of communication between them and the champions in different parts of the hospital must be maintained. The champions remain responsible for keeping an eye on their units, making sure there is no falling off in adherence to the bladder bundle, and alerting the project leaders to problems or potential problems. If one or another nurse or physician champion is about to be reassigned or plans to leave the hospital, for example, a replacement must be found. In fact, the executive sponsor suggests that the team should routinely urge current champions to develop potential replacements for themselves.

Of course, there will always be backsliders, those who revert to the old ways of doing things. A nurse shared with us her problem with a handful of physicians who have always, she said, thought along the lines of, "This patient is incontinent—of course they need a catheter." She defined her challenge in these terms: "It is changing their paradigm and making it stick. I can think I have them all headed in the right direction and then, six months later, I am back saying, 'Hey, what do you think about taking this catheter out?' with the same physician again."

The champions throughout the hospital will also be responsible for providing the infection prevention department with a once-a-week count of the Foleys in their units, a substantial easing of the daily catheter patrol that operated during the intervention. And each month, the infection preventionists will issue a report providing the current and past Foley prevalence and CAUTI rate for each of the hospital's units. It will be sent to all of the units as well as the hospital's administrative and clinical leadership and will be posted on the hospital's website.

The updated data will enable the members of each unit to measure their progress in the war on CAUTI. Because they are on the frontline of that struggle, and because the patients are so directly in their care, these reports are of particular concern to the nurses and nurse managers in the various departments. The intervention has succeeded in large measure because of their acceptance of the bladder bundle changes, and they have a professional and personal stake in preserving that achievement. Any report of an increase in Foley use or in the CAUTI rate is likely to spur them to take corrective action. It's their duty, yes, but it's also a matter of professional pride.

The monthly evaluations serve another purpose. They remind management that the CAUTI initiative carries on, albeit at a reduced level. That helps maintain C-suite support for the sustainability program and its personnel. It's never a good idea to allow your project to fall completely off the radar screen.

The leaders of the sustainability program at the model hospital are keenly aware of the inevitable arrival of new quality improvement projects, and of the time and resources these newcomers demand of clinicians—time and resources that might be stolen from the CAUTI prevention mission. Quality campaigns are so thick on the ground these days that they end up competing against each other. The members of the team are determined that their project will not be viewed as part of that competition. They want it to be seen as providing benefits for other safety efforts, as a potential partner in new interventions.

If a quality initiative to reduce pressure ulcers appears at the hospital, for instance, the CAUTI prevention team will link to it, pointing out that

Foleys tend to keep patients immobile and more susceptible to the ulcers. Thus, both the pressure ulcer and CAUTI projects share the goal of using Foleys only when medically necessary and removing them as soon as possible. The CAUTI prevention effort can also be linked to the Surgical Care Improvement Project (SCIP), which focuses on significantly reducing surgical complications. Because the absence of a Foley in postoperative patients allows for their greater mobility, it can also promote more rapid recovery.

One challenge to the sustainability of the CAUTI prevention initiative will be the arrival of new physicians and nurses at the hospital, people who may not be familiar with the requirements of the bladder bundle. To prepare for this, the team leaders will make sure that online CAUTI prevention instruction and other educational materials are part of the hospital's orientation process, and they assure each unit champion that they stand ready to help if there are problems with any newcomers. The director of a medical intensive care unit who was sustaining a CLABSI prevention initiative described the orientation process: "That's like an ongoing thing. . . . People coming in from hospitals across the country who aren't doing this. They're learning a whole new system, so it's kind of intense training. Everybody up to speed all the time."

That process is somewhat eased by the fact that the new arrivals are often younger and more open to fresh ideas than their predecessors. "It is hard to teach an old dog new tricks," an infection preventionist told us with some satisfaction, "but with a new puppy it is easy."

Openness to change, the project leaders recognize, should also apply to the post-intervention period as a whole. Sustainability should not equal entrenchment. The champions should always be alert to any possible improvements that can be made to the ways they support and promote the initiative. Should the Foley data be gathered more often—or less often? Is there a better way to remind bedside nurses of the availability of alternatives to the Foley? Is the patient education material doing the job?

Such questions are on the agenda at the monthly sustainability meetings of the project leaders. They also review the latest data from the infection prevention department, looking for changes in Foley prevalence. And they take up any problems that have arisen since the previous session and discuss possible solutions. Yes, the items in the bladder bundle have become second nature for most of the model hospital's clinicians, but there are always a few backsliders to keep track of and a few newcomers to watch out for—and the need to help one or another unit champion find a replacement. At a meeting of the leaders of a quality improvement project committed to sustaining change, there's always something to talk about.

The experience at one hospital is instructive. An intervention there reduced the number of inappropriate catheters to nearly zero—and cut CAUTI rates by 39%.[1] To sustain these advances, the hospital continued to use, as part of routine nursing care, a computerized nursing template for assessing which patients on each shift had a catheter and whether that catheter met appropriateness criteria. If the catheter was considered inappropriate, it would be removed. As part of the effort to hardwire the intervention, physicians received a monthly e-mail message from the chief of medicine to remind them that CAUTI prevention continued to be a priority and to reiterate his support for having the nurses essentially be stewards of the urinary catheters. The name of the physician champion was displayed in the e-mail in case other physicians had questions. Finally, monitoring of important outcomes, such as the proportion of catheters that were appropriate and the CAUTI rates, continued. This data was shared with the frontline staff as well as with others in the organization. The results of this approach were impressive: Three years after the CAUTI prevention initiative began, the hospital recorded a 12-month period with just a single CAUTI.

MAINTAINING PROGRESS IN HAND HYGIENE

Among the most urgent sustainability goals, in general, is the effort to maintain progress in improving hospitals' hand hygiene practices. Perhaps the single most important cause of healthcare-associated infection is the widespread failure of healthcare workers to follow proper handwashing procedures. We participated in hand hygiene sustainability studies at hospital units in Florence, Italy, where we saw how an intervention's substantial progress in improving hand hygiene could be sustained over a four-year period in one unit—and how another unit's adherence to the handwashing protocol plummeted after the hand hygiene champion left his leadership post.[2]

In the unit with stable leadership, adherence held at 71% compared to 37% before the intervention began. In the unit that lost its champion, adherence dropped among nurses from 51% to 8%. Among physicians, the fall was from 51% to 3%! An active leadership and team effort are key elements in sustaining any quality improvement.

In another sustainability study,[3] this one following up on Michigan's Keystone ICU intervention, the much-reduced rates of CLABSI at the end of the intervention were maintained and even further reduced after 18 months. During interviews at the participating hospitals, ICU team members pointed to the continuous feedback of infection data and the active involvement and support of senior leadership as major contributors to sustainability. The feedback provided the team with a kind of report card on their efforts, alerting them to any increase in infection or offering proof that CLABSI was still under control.

In the next chapter, as promised, we describe the collaborative option, the joining of a group of hospitals to pursue a specific quality improvement initiative. It is an alternative to the single-hospital model we have focused on up to this point. Collaboratives have become extremely popular, particularly in efforts to prevent healthcare-associated infection. They may be a good option for some hospitals, but they do have their drawbacks.

SUGGESTIONS FOR FURTHER READING

di Martino, P., Ban, K. M., Bartoloni, A., Fowler, K. E., Saint, S., & Mannelli, F. (2011). Assessing the sustainability of hand hygiene adherence prior to patient contact in the emergency department: A 1-year post-intervention evaluation. *American Journal of Infection Control, 39*(1), 14–18.

In this study, the authors assess the sustainability of a previously published, successful hand hygiene intervention in a pediatric emergency department in Florence, Italy. They found that compliance one year after the initiative (~45%) was consistent with that immediately post-intervention (~45%). Their data also showed that there was an increase in adherence over this time among nurses (41% to 50%) and a marked decrease among physicians (50% to 36%). These results indicate the differences that can develop between healthcare providers during a sustainability program.

Fakih, M. G., Rey, J. E., Pena, M. E., Szpunar, S., & Saravolatz, L. D. (2013). Sustained reductions in urinary catheter use over 5 years: Bedside nurses view themselves responsible for evaluation of catheter necessity. *American Journal of Infection Control, 41*, 236–239.

In this study of non-ICUs at an 800-bed tertiary-care teaching hospital in Michigan, the authors evaluate the effect of a multimodal intervention to increase appropriate urinary catheter use and the ability to sustain that compliance. During the five years of the study, there was a significant reduction in urinary catheter use from 17.3% to 12.7% ($p<.0001$).

Lieber, S. R., Mantengoli, E., Saint, S., Fowler, K. E., Fumagalli, C., Bartolozzi, D., ... Bartoloni, A. (2014). The effect of leadership on hand hygiene: Assessing hand hygiene adherence prior to patient contact in 2 infectious disease units in Tuscany. *Infection Control and Hospital Epidemiology, 35*(3), 313–316.

In this study of an infectious diseases unit at a hospital in Florence, Italy, Lieber and colleagues assessed the sustainability of a successful multimodal hand hygiene initiative over four years. They found that hand hygiene adherence among all healthcare workers was significantly higher 4 years after the intervention (71%) compared with pre-intervention rates (37%). A study of another infectious diseases unit that had not participated in the intervention but was under the direction of the intervention's physician champion, demonstrated a significant drop in adherence among nurses (51% to 8%) and among physicians (51% to 3%) after he retired. The results of this study illustrate the success of the intervention as well as the effects of leadership on hand hygiene practices.

Matar, D. S., Pham, J. C., Louis, T. A., & Berenholtz, S. M. (2013). Achieving and sustaining ventilator-associated pneumonia-free time among intensive care units (ICUs): Evidence from the Keystone ICU Quality Improvement Collaborative. *Infection Control and Hospital Epidemiology, 34*(7), 740–743.

This retrospective analysis of the Michigan Keystone ICU collaborative demonstrated that adult ICUs could achieve and sustain a zero rate of ventilator-associated pneumonia (VAP) for a considerable number of ventilator and calendar months. Half of the participating ICUs achieved 26.2 consecutive VAP-free ventilator-months. And in terms of calendar months, half of the ICUs went over 6 months and three-quarters of the ICUs went nearly 12 months without a case of VAP. These results have important public health implications and can inform realistic best-practice benchmarks.

Stirman, S. W., Kimberly, J., Cook, N., Calloway, A., Castro, F. & Charns, M. (2012). The sustainability of new programs and innovations: A review of the empirical literature and recommendations for future research. *Implementation Science, 7*, 17.

In this review of the research literature, the authors evaluated 125 studies related to sustainability. They found that most published studies are retrospective and approximately half rely on self-reported data. They are equally divided between quantitative and qualitative methods, and few of them employ rigorous methods of evaluation. Research in this area is lacking in respect to the extent, nature, and impact of adaptations to the interventions or programs once implemented. The results of this search suggest that while prospective and experimental designs are needed, there is also an important role for qualitative research in efforts to understand the phenomenon, refine hypotheses, and develop strategies to promote sustainment.

The Collaborative Approach
to Preventing Infection

A single arrow is easily broken but not ten in a bundle.

—JAPANESE PROVERB

His hospital, along with dozens of others, had just participated in a quality improvement collaborative, and the infection prevention tionist was impressed—to a degree. For years, he had tried, and failed, to convince the attending physicians to update their approach to central lines. "If nothing else," he said, "this project has been instrumental in getting that change to happen. Before, it was me fighting the wolves."

Yet the infection preventionist was dissatisfied with the project's overall impact. It had the vocal support of the hospital's top officials, he explained, "but we never got the backing monetarily or time-wise." Even though many staff members wanted to participate, they were not allowed to take time away from their regular duties, so the collaborative became "just another one of those things," as he put it, just another in a long list of demanding quality improvement initiatives.

A similar ambivalence can be found in many studies of collaboratives. Even as this communal approach to enhancing healthcare has been taken up by more and more hospitals across the country, and won support from federal agencies and dozens of state governments, questions remain about its effectiveness. There are a variety of collaborative models, but in this chapter we look at the operation of a generic quality improvement collaborative, particularly those aspects that differ from the kind of single-hospital initiative described in the previous chapters. We also suggest how a hospital and its project team can make the most of the collaborative experience.

JAPANESE BEGINNINGS

The history of the quality improvement collaborative can be traced back to the 1980s and the emergence of the continuous improvement process in Japan. As preached by Kaoru Ishikawa and W. Edwards Deming, the continuous improvement process assumes that you can endlessly improve a manufacturing process by continuously gathering and evaluating feedback about how the process is actually working out, and then applying what you've learned to improve the process. This program of incremental improvement is central to Kaizen, the practice that helped Toyota revolutionize automotive manufacturing worldwide.

The feedback mechanism was eventually adapted to the needs of healthcare with the routine collection and analysis of data about patients and medical outcomes as a path toward better treatment options. That technique is a staple of today's quality improvement collaboratives.

The emergence of this movement is generally credited to the lackluster quality improvement record of individual hospitals. Pressure had been mounting, from governments and the public, for hospitals to improve their clinical results and to control spiraling costs. The collaborative was seen as a means to both ends, in part by imposing an external discipline on participating institutions. It no doubt also benefited from the universal perception that there is, as Homer put it so many eons ago, "strength in unity."

Over the centuries, that concept has served many different kinds of masters. The strengththroughunity.org website, for example, is dedicated to the rebuilding of a Haitian area devastated by the 2010 hurricane. More ominously, the concept was central to the National Fascist Party, which ruled Italy from 1922 to 1943. The party took its name from the Latin word *fascis,* or *bundle,* and used a cylinder of birch rods as its symbol; any single rod might easily be broken, but the bundle of rods would endure. By extension, it was hoped that the binding of a number of hospitals into a collaborative would yield a stronger performance than that achieved by individual hospitals. The bundle theory has another application in these pages, of course: The complete set of practices within the bladder bundle has a stronger impact than would those practices implemented separately.

A COLLABORATIVE AT THE MODEL HOSPITAL

Our look at a relatively generic quality improvement collaborative starts early one Monday morning when the CEO of our model hospital learns that a national agency is putting together a country-wide collaborative aimed at reducing catheter-associated urinary tract infection (CAUTI). The model hospital is on its list of intended participants. The CEO asks his top clinical people to consider whether the hospital should take part, and eventually calls for a meeting to discuss the matter.

Collaborative sponsors choose their topic with care, since it can determine the project's success or failure. The topic needs to be broad enough to appeal to a hospital's administration as important and marketable— yet narrow enough to require no more than a reasonable investment of time and energy on the part of the hospital's staff. It needs to be evidence-based and scientific—yet not so technically complicated that it will be difficult to learn. Above all, the topic should require a positive change—but not so much of a change that it will inspire widespread clinical resistance.

At the meeting called by the model hospital's CEO, the chief medical officer—having never read the preceding chapters—reports that the hospital's CAUTI rate is considerably higher than it should be. Both he and the chief nursing executive express concern about the staff time and resources a collaborative would require, especially given the current high number of quality improvement initiatives at the hospital. The CEO acknowledges that argument, but he points out that the sponsoring national agency carries professional and financial clout that can make it difficult for hospitals to ignore an invitation to join the collaborative. In fact, the agency actually supports some of the model hospital's own quality improvement programs. And the CEO recognizes the need to reduce healthcare-associated infection (HAI)—as a medical matter, as a marketing matter now that these statistics are publicly on display, and as a financial imperative since the Centers for Medicare & Medicaid Services stopped reimbursing hospitals for many HAIs. He also doesn't want to be odd man out, refusing to join the collaborative if his peers at nearby hospitals sign on. After weighing all the benefits and challenges, he decides to join the collaborative effort. The CEO asks the chief nurse to take it over.

To serve as the sponsor, leading the model hospital's participation in the collaborative, the chief nurse chooses her deputy, the director of nursing—who, in turn, selects as project manager the unit manager of a first-rate inpatient nursing unit. A physician champion and a nurse champion are then recruited, along with the infection preventionist, completing the core membership of the project team. (The core membership of the CAUTI prevention team was discussed in Table 4.1 of Chapter 4.)

Though it takes just a few sentences here, the selection of the team's sponsor, leadership, and composition has actually been a careful and somewhat lengthy process. The chief nurse understands that the intervention is a complex and inherently difficult project, the participants driven by a variety of sometimes conflicting motives. Those devoted to advancing their careers, for example, may be more interested in the chance to meet with clinicians from other hospitals and the leadership title than in the responsibilities that go with that title. The CEO may be more eager to show the hospital's flag than to properly finance the initiative. The chief nurse knows that if the team leaders are not willing to work within the requirements and discipline of the collaborative, the project is doomed from the start.

AN 18-MONTH PROJECT GETS UNDERWAY

At the statewide kick-off meeting, the core team from the model hospital and teams from dozens of other hospitals meet the faculty experts from various professional societies who will be their instructors and mentors during the course of the collaboration. A representative from the sponsoring agency lays out the essentials of the 18-month-long project: The widespread impact of CAUTI on patients, the scientific evidence behind the bladder bundle, the importance of removing inappropriate Foleys, and, in particular, the need to gain the cooperation of bedside nurses and other frontline staff. They may have good reason to be resistant because of the extra demands of the initiative on their time, especially if there have been several recent in-house quality projects. There will be more educational sessions before the actual intervention begins, and regularly scheduled telephone and in-person meetings. The collaborative is designed to maximize these learning interactions—it is an important component of the project's "strength in unity."

In all their early presentations, the experts ask the model hospital and the other participants to plan their initiatives with long-term sustainability in mind. The processes that will be changed during the implementation should be hardwired into the hospital's operations from the get-go—the CAUTI prevention nursing template should be understood to be a permanent addition, for example, and that should be true of the monitoring of Foley rates as well. The project leaders and champions should be selected for the long term: Are they the kind of people who will ensure that the benefits of the initiative will live on once the collaborative has run its course?

Each hospital's project leaders will have to arrange for a baseline assessment of indwelling urinary catheters and the incidence of CAUTI, and maintain a daily record of that data throughout the implementation. The baseline data and a monthly update will be shared with the managers of the collaborative. During the planning phase, there will be calls every other week with extra time devoted to sessions on how to collect, organize, and analyze these data and on processes that have proven to be a major stumbling block for earlier collaborative teams.

During these group calls, experts offer advice and answer questions. In this way, as they exchange ideas, a sense of community forms and a behavioral norm evolves. The educational efforts also include a website with transcripts of the educational sessions and answers to frequently asked questions, as well as regular webinars that feature discussions of the project's basics and of implementation challenges—along with possible solutions—that have come up at several sites.

Once the actual implementation begins, all teams, regardless of how far along they are in the project, are required to take part in two calls each month, one state and one national. The calls are informal and interactive, providing opportunities for teams to share their experiences and help each other overcome problems. Each team is also expected to provide monthly electronic reports of its CAUTI data, keeping the collaborative leadership and other teams aware of everyone's progress—or lack of progress. New strategies are welcome: The project manager at the model hospital, for example, reports on its program to have a nurse trained in the bladder bundle take part in multidisciplinary rounds, keeping an eye out for inappropriate Foleys and urging their removal if found; the program has led to a substantial drop in the rate of Foley use.

Social occasions are designed to build the teams' comfort level, relieving the feeling some team members have that they are alone in this challenging endeavor. The social encounters also build mutual trust, encouraging the teams to share experiences, including best practices. These gatherings occur during the three in-person learning sessions—at the kick-off, at the nine-month midway point, and at the end of the collaborative. Time is set aside during lunch and coffee breaks to allow teams to intermingle and interact. These "constructive collisions" are one of the key rationales for the in-person meetings.

The frontline activity in a quality improvement collaborative is similar to that found in a single-hospital initiative, and so are many of the problems including active resisters, organizational constipators, and timeservers. However, there are other potential difficulties that can arise because of the very structure of the collaborative. The team leaders at each hospital have presumably learned a great deal about preventing CAUTI, and in theory, that advice has been effectively communicated to the other members of the project team. In practice, though, that exchange of information is often inadequate. The communication failures occur in the opposite direction, as well, with bedside nurses failing to share the details of their problems with project team members and team members failing to report internal team problems to the project sponsor.

A COOKIE-CUTTER EXPERIENCE

By its very nature, the typical collaborative provides hospitals with a cookie-cutter experience. The educational materials and bladder bundles are identical for all hospitals, there is a common set of measures the teams track, and participants are expected to follow the same schedules and procedures. Team leaders do have some opportunity to air their particular problems and seek solutions but, given the collaborative's central direction, there is far less of the natural tailoring of a quality improvement project than can be found in most single-hospital initiatives.

Studies of quality improvement collaboratives have warned about a tendency on the part of organizers to focus on didactic talks, leaving little time for discussions of implementation problems at individual hospitals. Aware of this concern, the experts serving some collaboratives set aside hours for private meetings with teams that are having trouble and have little or no idea why. Some collaboratives have even created a special group, including a physician, nurse, and quality improvement expert, which is available to visit hospitals that are struggling with the implementation process. Usually the group responds to a request from such hospitals, though it sometimes will offer its assistance when a particular intervention is floundering or a hospital appears to be on the verge of dropping out of the collaborative. (By one estimate, up to 30% of hospitals in a collaborative leave the program before its conclusion.[1])

During their site visits, these experts interview a broad cross-section of the target hospital's staff, C-suite to bedside nurse, with particular attention paid to the project team members. Gradually a picture emerges of the hospital's culture, the staff's attitudes toward quality improvement interventions in general, and the roadblocks in the way of this intervention. The experts will then suggest ways to tailor the intervention to fit the local setting. Instead of promoting the bladder bundle as an all-or-nothing proposition, for example, the consultants may propose implementing only those practices that seem feasible given the hospital's context or culture. If the nurse-initiated Foley removal protocol is not tenable, the experts will offer other options—a computerized reminder for physicians, or prominent reminders on patients' charts. If a nurse manager is standing in the way of progress, the expert group will propose ways to bypass him. Sometimes a hospital that is unwilling to accept the adaptive aspects of a bundle will be more ready to buy a new piece of equipment.

Though the people overseeing the collaborative have no legal power over the laggard hospitals, they do have ways to prod them forward. The various interactions of the teams, built into the collaborative, create a pressure to live up to those teams with the most improved catheter rates. As one physician told us, the collaborative is "a big motivator for us to say, 'O.K., we're trying to get ourselves to the same standard as everyone else's standards.'" But that competitive pressure can have a negative impact as well, embarrassing laggard teams. In a study identifying the features that participants in 53 collaboratives found most helpful,[2] one hospital's project manager described the attitude some teams have toward the online interactions: "People just feel intimidated to use it because they don't want to ask a question that people will think is stupid."

The same study found that the sharing aspects of collaboratives such as solicitation of staff ideas and learning session interactions received fairly high ratings. Yet when the helpfulness of the interactive aspects was broken down between participating teams that improved significantly and those that did not, it showed that interaction received considerably higher helpfulness ratings among the more successful teams. "Our results suggest," the author said, "that collaboratives may work most for participants who capitalize on their interorganizational features in addition to their intra-organizational features."

On the face of it, the quality improvement collaborative appears to be a most reasonable approach to the refractory hospital infection problem. Indeed, many studies of collaboratives have reported substantial improvements in infection results, greatly reducing device-associated rates, for example. But systematic reviews of the quality improvement collaborative literature have raised questions, including some about the accuracy of the uncontrolled collaborative studies. As one commentator put it, "They were probably biased in favour of positive findings in successful teams."[3]

The systematic reviews have also found a disturbing lack of consistency in the collaborative outcomes. Why do so many hospitals drop out of collaboratives even though taking part in the same program as their peers? Why is the evidence of positive change on the provider level—in terms of medication management, for instance—generally not matched by evidence of comparable gains on the patient level? Why do so many of the hospitals that do well in collaboratives already have a strong, patient-centered, cooperative culture in place and a positive record of successful internal quality improvement initiatives?

THE ADVANTAGES OF A COLLABORATIVE

In general, a collaborative project is of greatest value to hospitals that have the desire to undertake a given quality improvement initiative but lack the tools and the expertise to go it on their own. They don't have to spend their own resources and staff time reinventing the wheel for an in-house quality intervention. A hospital considering a collaborative, however, should be prepared for the inevitable friction that occurs when an outside entity imposes its program on a medical institution.

The hospital's clinicians may be told to do things that are against current hospital policy: requiring the use of chlorhexidine, for example, or empowering bedside nurses to remove Foleys. The record of the hospital's success or failure in meeting the goals of the collaborative, month by month, will be widely broadcast among the participants. And if a hospital taking part in a collaborative does have some expertise in the particular initiative, the hospital should make sure those experts are working cooperatively with the outside experts or the whole project could be put at risk.

Discipline is central to the strength of any collaborative, and participating hospital teams must toe the line if the initiative is to succeed. The teams need to perform according to the collaborative leadership's directives. Hospitals that want initiatives that are shaped to fit their particular environment and culture are more likely to prefer running their own, in-house quality improvement projects.

In any event, the lack of a sufficient body of controlled studies of these collaboratives has made it difficult to judge their overall effectiveness. Without such scientific results, the reasons for participants' success or failure in implementing change and the particular aspects of collaboratives that lead teams to move in one or the other direction remain uncertain. Because the collaborative process itself is so complex and varies from one initiative to another, and because the institutions that participate in a collaborative are themselves so infinitely complex, a definitive scientific evaluation of their interaction has remained an unanswered challenge.

Thus far in the book, we have focused on examples of hospital infections that arise from the use of devices, such as catheters or ventilators. But as we noted in Chapter 1, our approach to gaining the cooperation of clinicians in the adoption of preventive interventions can serve as a model for other important hospital initiatives such as preventing pressure ulcers or falls. In the next chapter, we show how that might play out in an initiative aimed at preventing *Clostridium difficile* infection, an increasingly common hazard of hospitalization.

SUGGESTIONS FOR FURTHER READING

The Breakthrough Series: IHI's collaborative model for achieving breakthrough improvement. (2003). IHI Innovation Series white paper. Boston, MA: Institute for Healthcare Improvement.

This white paper presents an overview of the successful collaborative approach that the Institute for Healthcare Improvement (IHI) has developed to improve healthcare by supporting change. With the experience of over 50 collaboratives, the study reports on the tested and refined Breakthrough Series model, which offers a framework for bringing about dramatic and lasting change.

Fakih, M. G., George, C., Edson, B. S., Goeschel, C. A., & Saint, S. (2013). Implementing a national program to reduce catheter-associated urinary tract infection: A quality improvement collaboration of state hospital associations, academic medical centers, professional societies, and governmental agencies. *Infection Control and Hospital Epidemiology, 34*(10), 1048–1054.

In this article, the authors present an overview of the national effort to reduce the risk of catheter-associated urinary tract infection (CAUTI), funded by the Agency for Healthcare Research and Quality. Based on the successful pilot work in Michigan led by the Michigan Health and Hospital Association Keystone Center, the project has the following key components: (1) centralized coordination of the effort and dissemination of information, (2) data collection based on established definitions and approaches, (3) focused guidance on the technical practices that will prevent CAUTI, (4) emphasis on understanding the socio-adaptive aspects, and (5) partnering with specialty organizations and governmental agencies that have expertise in the relevant subject area.

Nembhard, I. M. (2009). Learning and improving in quality improvement collaboratives: Which collaborative features do participants value most? *Health Services Research, 44*(Part 1), 359–378.

Using surveys and semistructured interviews, the author identifies features that participants in various collaborations supported by the Institute for Healthcare Improvement (IHI) found most helpful for advancing improvement efforts overall and knowledge acquisition in particular. Nembhard's findings identify features of collaborative design and implementation that participants view as most helpful, including interorganizational features.

Saint, S., Greene, M. T, Kowalski, C. P., Watson, S. R., Hofer, T. P., & Krein, S. L. (2013). Preventing catheter-associated urinary tract infection in the United States: A national comparative study. *JAMA Internal Medicine, 173*(10), 874–879.

In this study, the authors conducted a survey of 470 infection preventionists to compare the use of specific infection prevention practices by U.S. hospitals. Their results showed that Michigan hospitals, compared with hospitals in the rest of the United States, more frequently participated in collaboratives to reduce HAIs (94% versus 67%), which may have contributed to the fact that Michigan hospitals had a 25% reduction in the rate of CAUTIs (compared to 6% reduction in the rest of the United States).

Taking on *C. Difficile*

All diseases begin in the gut.

—HIPPOCRATES

B etween July 1, 1986, and July 31, 1987, the staff of a Veterans Affairs Healthcare System in Minnesota conducted an active surveillance of cases of diarrhea associated with the bacterium, *Clostridium difficile*.[1] The initiative was part of a controlled trial to determine how the use of vinyl gloves in dealing with all body substances would affect the incidence of life-threatening *C. difficile* infection. To help convince hospital personnel in the two test wards to use the gloves, the goals of the trial were promoted with posters and in-service programs. Boxes of gloves were placed next to every bed. The result: In the wards with the gloves, the incidence of infection plummeted from 7.7 cases per 1,000 patient discharges during the six months before the initiative to 1.5 cases per 1,000 discharges during the six-month-long prevention program. The incidence in the two control wards was unchanged.

In other words, more than a quarter of a century ago, some hospitals were finding effective ways to control *C. difficile*. Yet over the decades since then, its incidence has soared. Between 2000 and 2009, hospital cases of the infection rose from 139,000 to 336,000.[2] Its death toll, including nursing homes as well as hospitals, has shot up to more than 14,000 Americans a year as a new, more virulent strain has spread far and wide across North America and Europe.

For reasons both technical and socio-adaptive, hospital initiatives to cope with *C. difficile* have frequently fallen short. There is a lack of randomized, gold-standard studies to support a number of the current best practices used to prevent and control the infection, which has led some hospital personnel to oppose quality interventions based upon those practices. The *C. difficile* prevention bundle also requires difficult behavioral changes. In fact, though *C. difficile* and catheter-associated urinary tract infection (CAUTI) are very different, the adaptive aspects are similar in many ways. In this chapter, we show how the adaptive approach of the previous chapters on CAUTI can be applied to *C. difficile* prevention.

THE NATURE OF *C. DIFFICILE*

The *C. difficile* bacterium produces spores that enter the outer world through feces; they can survive for months or years on surfaces such as hands and bedding and can easily become airborne, landing on food and drink. When they find their way back into a human intestine, the spores mature into new *C. difficile* bacteria. Small-scale colonization of the bacteria in the gut usually produces no symptoms, but large numbers can lead to an infection, producing abdominal pain, intestinal inflammation, and diarrhea. The infection generally strikes those who have been exposed to *C. difficile* in a hospital or nursing home and those who have taken broad-spectrum antimicrobials; these powerful drugs can wipe out the normal healthy bacteria residing in the gastrointestinal tract allowing *C. difficile* to flourish and cause infection. Old age is another risk factor—10 times greater for people 65 and older than for younger people.[3] And once a person has the infection, the chance of a recurrence can be as high as 20%.

C. difficile is a major public health problem. The Centers for Disease Control and Prevention has found that 75% of *C. difficile* infection appeared in people who were not hospitalized at the time, though that group was mainly made up of people recently hospitalized, outpatients, and those who were residents in nursing homes. There is also growing concern that carriers of *C. difficile* who are asymptomatic may be a much more important source of the infection than previously believed—that a colonized but symptom-free nurse or grandchild may cause *C. difficile* infection simply by spending time in the room of a patient who is on an antimicrobial. A British study using molecular typing actually found that, "in a majority of cases, *C. difficile* infection is not transmitted from another symptomatic patient."[4]

When the administrative and medical leaders at our model, 250-bed hospital decide to pursue a *C. difficile* initiative, they are responding to some of the same pressures they faced with their CAUTI initiative. The hospital's infection rate is too high, increasing the risk for patients. In 2013, *C. difficile* was added to the list of healthcare-associated infections whose rates hospitals must report to the Centers for Medicare & Medicaid Services (CMS) for public posting so that a high rate can be a marketing problem. There are some direct financial concerns as well. In 2015, *C. difficile* will join CAUTI on the list of HAIs that are not reimbursed when acquired in the hospital. Infection with *C. difficile* increases the average hospital stay by 2.6 to 4.5 days, and each episode costs hospitals an estimated $2,470 to $3,669.[5] Infection with *C. difficile* may also, in the not too distant future, join CAUTI and other infections as the target of a program that trims overall CMS payments to the worst performers in reducing hospital-acquired conditions.

CREATING A *C. DIFFICILE* BUNDLE

At the model hospital, the C-suite agrees that a *C. difficile* prevention bundle should be created along the CAUTI lines, and that a CAUTI-like team should be formed to run the initiative. There will, however, be important differences in the team membership, the scope of the initiative, and the elements of the bundle. In the case of CAUTI, for example, clinicians were asked to limit their use of a Foley to a much-reduced list of indications and to remove the catheter as soon as medically appropriate. In a *C. difficile* prevention initiative, perhaps the single essential requirement on the to-do list is for heightened stewardship of broad-spectrum antimicrobials. The drugs increase a person's chance of developing *C. difficile* infection by 7 to 10 times while taking the drugs and for a month thereafter, and they are frequently prescribed inappropriately.[2] In a study at a nursing home in Rhode Island,[6] more than 40% of the patients were found to have been given antimicrobials unnecessarily. Based on their study of patients from 183 hospitals who had been given antimicrobials during their stay, the authors of a recent report estimated that a 30% reduction in broad-spectrum antimicrobials will lead to a 26% cut in *C. difficile* infection.[7] As we shall see, antimicrobial restrictions do not always sit well with physicians and nurses—or with patients and their families. (See Box 9.1.)

ASSEMBLING THE TEAM

The model hospital's *C. difficile* prevention team, like the CAUTI prevention team, has a multidisciplinary makeup, including someone from senior leadership, a project manager, physician and nurse champions, an infection preventionist, and laboratory personnel. But there are some important early additions to the team. They include a manager from environmental services to coordinate room cleaning and an inpatient pharmacist who will be a key figure in antimicrobial stewardship.

One of the team's first decisions concerns the scope of the intervention. The CAUTI project team chose to follow the path of caution, testing and improving a pilot initiative before scaling up. But there are compelling reasons for the *C. difficile* prevention team to start big. Antimicrobial stewardship is inherently a hospital-wide mission, and some elements of the *C. difficile* prevention bundle—special room-cleaning directions, for example—can be more efficiently coped with on a full-scale basis.

Box 9.1   ADAPTED FROM FLANDERS & SAINT[8]

Like many drugs, antimicrobials have the potential to both benefit and harm the patient for whom they are prescribed. Unique to antimicrobials, however, is the potential to harm others because of the spread of *C. difficile* and because the excessive use of antimicrobials has created a host of deadly antimicrobial-resistant bacteria. Thus, prescribing antimicrobials for a patient with a possible bacterial infection—who may or may not benefit from their use—requires a physician to weigh the potential benefit for the patient against the potential harm to the patient and society.[9] This long-standing tension is a manifestation, at least in part, of an even longer-standing battle played out between the political philosophies of John Locke and Jean-Jacques Rousseau.

As one of the authors noted in a recent essay in JAMA Internal Medicine,[8] Locke—a 17th-century British physician whose theories influenced America's Founding Fathers—believed in the importance of the individual as "free and equal" and in the individual's right to make decisions based on his own judgment and beliefs. In order to best protect themselves and their property, individuals form a body politic, thereby agreeing to certain standards of behavior. Self-interest leads people to form governments; however, individuals may dissolve their government if it ceases to work solely in their best interest. In short, government has no sovereignty of its own.

Jean-Jacques Rousseau, an influential 18th-century European philosopher argued that the "general will"—a collectively held will that prioritizes the common interest—is far more important than individual will. Writing in *The Social Contract*, Rousseau argued: "... whoever refuses to obey the general will shall be compelled to do so by the whole body. This means nothing less than that he will be forced to be free ... "[10]

The tension between advantaging society or the individual plays out daily when physicians decide whether to prescribe antimicrobials in the hospital. More often than not, the interest of the individual prevails and antimicrobials are prescribed. This, in part, reflects

(continued)

Box 9.1 (Continued)

a very strong desire on the part of clinicians to avoid the chagrin
associated with withholding antimicrobials in a patient ultimately
found to have a bacterial infection.[11] So in these daily battles, the
emphasis on individualism espoused by Locke appears to rule
the day. As a result, there has been little progress in reducing
antimicrobial overuse.

Antimicrobial stewardship is a quality initiative unto itself, addressing a range of issues not limited to C. *difficile* prevention. The project
team examines the hospital's current policies for prescribing antimicrobials—and finds it wanting. The hospital epidemiologist and pharmacist design a new protocol that rules out the use of two high-risk,
broad-spectrum antimicrobials on patients at high-risk for developing
C. *difficile* infection unless a first-line drug is not available, and the protocol wins C-suite approval. The order is then widely distributed within
the hospital, and occasional reminders are issued during the course of
the intervention.

The team also considers other options, including a requirement that
no prescription for the two antimicrobials be filled without the approval
of either the hospital epidemiologist or the pharmacist. The decision is
made to adopt a more prospective approach. After filling a prescription
for a broad-spectrum antimicrobial, pharmacists will review the patient's
chart to determine whether the drug is appropriate. If not, the hospital
epidemiologist (who is also an infectious diseases physician) will contact
the prescribing physician to discuss the issue.

PROTECTIVE MEASURES

The model hospital's C. *difficile* prevention bundle emphasizes the need
for clinicians to use protective measures to halt the spread of infection

once prevention has failed. They are to wear gloves when handling any and all patients' feces. They are to observe full barrier precautions, including gloves and gowns for all visitors to the patient and meticulous hand hygiene with soap and water after glove removal. (Some studies have shown that alcohol-based cleansers are not effective against *C. difficile*.) Patient equipment will not be shared. Infected patients are to be housed in private rooms. After patients depart, their rooms are to be decontaminated with a solution containing household bleach, which has proven effective in killing *C. difficile* spores.

Just as the urinary tract infection rate is collected in a CAUTI initiative, the hospital's precise *C. difficile* infection rate pre-intervention will be measured as a baseline, and it will be monitored daily throughout the project. That process is complicated by the fact that a diagnostic test may be positive for a patient who is actually asymptomatic. The test data must be judged alongside the patient's symptoms: Is she suffering from diarrhea? Is she, or has she, recently been on antimicrobials? From a clinical standpoint, it is vital that the infection be quickly identified so that the patient can be isolated, both to prevent the spread of the infection and to begin treatment. The model hospital has empowered nurses, trained in the process, to speed up the identification by sending a watery stool to the lab for testing without waiting for a physician order.

Before the actual intervention begins, the project manager arranges for the education of the team members and the hospital as a whole about the risk factors for *C. difficile*, the ways in which it spreads, and the elements of the *C. difficile* prevention bundle to prevent and contain infection. Both in-person and online educational approaches are used. There are several meetings at which the responsibilities of the various team members are discussed.

The team members are also alerted to some of the reasons that clinicians and staff members might resist one or more parts of the bundle. Like the CAUTI intervention resisters, the project manager warns, there will be staff members who simply find the proposed changes inconvenient. People from environmental services, for example, may object to using bleach cleansers because of the unpleasant odor. Physicians may accept the items supported by A-level evidence but bridle at the less well-supported mandates such as the wearing of gowns, and some of them will surely object to having their prescriptions second-guessed. In general, doctors don't like to be told how to practice medicine.

The bundle provides clinicians with a checklist of requirements for preventing *C. difficile*, and once the actual intervention begins, the project manager sees to it that a copy of that list shows up on the patient's paper and electronic charts. Reminders are issued for those clinicians who resist, and posters listing the relevant parts of the bundle are placed in prominent locations in all of the hospital's clinical areas. (See Table 9.1.)

Patients and their families are informed about the infection and the initiative, seeking their cooperation in preventing its occurrence and its spread. They are encouraged to speak up if a nurse or physician fails to obey any of the bundle's injunctions. They are also asked not to lean on their physician to prescribe a broad-spectrum antimicrobial because it can so easily bring on *C. difficile* infection.

The good communications among the members of the project team, established before the start of the intervention, make it possible to cope with the inevitable unexpected problems. The project manager appeals to the executive sponsor for fresh funds to satisfy the sudden demand for supplies such as gloves and gowns and to provide overtime pay for the understaffed environmental services crew, now facing extra cleaning demands. Nurses appeal to the physician champion to have a heart-to-heart talk with an attending physician who regularly neglects to wash her hands with soap and water after examining a patient with *C. difficile*, instead relying on the alcohol-based hand rub that she routinely uses with other patients.

The infection preventionist on the team makes sure that the surveillance data is regularly dispatched to the team members, the hospital administration, and the various clinical units, where it serves as a goad to improve participation in the intervention and as evidence of progress in combating the infection.

Once their stool is normal, patients are typically released from the hospital while still on antimicrobial therapy to treat the *C. difficile* infection.

TABLE 9.1 C. DIFFICILE CHECKLIST (ADAPTED FROM ABBETT ET AL.[12])

Clostridium difficile Infection (CDI) Checklist

Hospital interventions to decrease the incidence and mortality of healthcare-associated C. _difficile_ infections

Prevention Checklist

- **When an MD, PA, NP, or RN suspects a patient has CDI:**

Physician, Physician Assistant, or Nurse Practitioner:

- Initiate _Contact Precautions Plus_
- Order stool C. _difficile_ toxin testing
- Discontinue nonessential antimicrobials
- Discontinue all antiperistaltic medications

Registered Nurse:

- Obtain stool sample for C. _difficile_ diagnostic test
- Place patient in single-patient room
- Place _Contact Precautions Plus_ sign on patient's door
- Ensure that gloves and gowns are easily accessible from patient's room
- Place dedicated stethoscope in patient's room
- Remind staff to wash hands with soap and water following patient contact

Treatment Checklist

- **When an MD, PA, or NP diagnoses mild CDI:** _All_ of the following criteria are present: diarrhea (<6 BM/day), no fever, WBC<15,000, no peritoneal signs, and no evidence of sepsis

Physician, Physician Assistant, or Nurse Practitioner:

- Initiate oral metronidazole at dose 500mg every 8 hours
- If no clinical improvement by 48–72 hours after diagnosis, treat patient as moderate CDI
- Continue therapy for at least 14 days total and at least 10 days after symptoms have abated

(continued)

TABLE 9.1 (Continued)

Clostridium difficile Infection (CDI) Checklist

Hospital interventions to decrease the incidence and mortality of healthcare-associated C. *difficile* infections

Prevention Checklist

Treatment Checklist

Microbiology Laboratory Staff Person:

- Call relevant patient floor with positive C. *difficile* toxin test result
- Provide daily list of positive test results for Infection Control

Infection Control Practitioner:

- Check microbiology results daily for positive C. *difficile* test results
- Call relevant floor to confirm that patient with positive C. *difficile* toxin results is in a single-patient room and that the *Contact Precautions Plus* sign is on the patient's door
- Flag the patient's C. *difficile* status in the hospital's clinical information system or in the patient's paper chart
- Alert housekeeping that the patient is on *Contact Precautions Plus*

When an MD, PA, or NP diagnoses moderate CDI:

At least one of the following criteria is present: diarrhea (6-12 BM/day), fever 37.5-38.5°C, WBC 15,000–25,000, or frankly visible stable lower gastrointestinal bleeding

Physician, Physician Assistant, or Nurse Practitioner:

- Initiate oral vancomycin at dose 250mg every 6 hours
- If no clinical improvement by 48 hours, add IV metronidazole at dose 500mg every 8 hours
- Consider obtaining infectious diseases consultation
- Consider obtaining abdominal CT scan
- Continue therapy for at least 14 days total and at least 10 days after symptoms have abated

TABLE 9.1 (Continued)

Clostridium difficile Infection (CDI) Checklist

Hospital interventions to decrease the incidence and mortality of healthcare-associated C. *difficile* infections

Prevention Checklist

Environmental Services Staff Person:

- Prior to discharge cleaning, check for *Contact Precautions Plus* sign on the patient's door

- If *Contact Precautions Plus* sign is on the door, clean the room with a bleach-based cleaning agent

- Confirm for supervisor that bleach-based cleaning agent was used for discharge cleaning for every patient on *Contact Precautions Plus*

Treatment Checklist

- **When an MD, PA, or NP diagnoses severe CDI:** *At least one* of the following criteria is present: diarrhea (>12 BM/day), fever >38.5°C, WBC >25,000, hemodynamic instability, marked & continuous abdominal pain, ileus, absence of bowel sounds, evidence of sepsis, or intensive care unit level of care required

Physician, Physician Assistant, or Nurse Practitioner:

- Obtain immediate infectious diseases consultation

- Obtain immediate general surgery consultation

- Obtain abdominal CT scan

- Initiate oral vancomycin at dose 250mg every 6 hours together with IV metronidazole at dose 500mg every 6 hours

- Following consultation with general surgery regarding its use, consider rectal vancomycin

- Ask general surgery service to assess the need for colectomy

Abbreviations: MD = medical doctor, PA = physician assistant, NP = nurse practitioner, RN = registered nurse, BM = bowel movement, WBC = white blood cell count, CT = computed tomography, IV = intravenous.

At the model hospital, prior to discharge, these patients are counseled to continue following the bundle directions at home, washing with soap and water and using bathroom cleansers containing bleach.

Throughout the intervention, the team leaders are alert to special circumstances that may require adjustments to elements of the bundle, either because of the nature of the patient population, for example, or because one or another element conflicts with established hospital policy. The CAUTI-type approach leaves room for interventions to be tailored to the particular needs or concerns of the individual hospital.

NEW TREATMENTS

A number of new treatments for *C. difficile* are being tested. The procedure that has attracted the most public attention calls for the infusion of donor feces in patients with recurrent *C. difficile* infection. In one study, diarrhea stopped after the first fecal infusion for 13 of the 16 patients; diarrhea was resolved in two of the remaining three patients after a second infusion from another donor.[13] Researchers have also successfully used nontoxigenic monoclonal antibodies to build up patients' resistance to toxigenic *C. difficile* and prevent a recurrence of the infection. Immunotherapy may eventually lead the way to a vaccine to prevent *C. difficile* infection among patients who are at high risk.

In the following chapter, we examine some of the new approaches, both technical and adaptive, that are being explored in the effort to reduce hospital infections. Meanwhile, though, too many hospital interventions to combat *C. difficile* in particular and healthcare-associated infection in general are achieving only modest results today. We believe that the adaptive approach described in this and earlier chapters can be applied to a substantial range of medical conditions to significantly improve those results.

SUGGESTIONS FOR FURTHER READING

Abbett, S. K., Yokoe, D. S., Lipsitz, S. R., Badar, A. M., Berry, W. R., Tamplin, E. M., & Gawande, A. A. (2009). Proposed checklist of hospital interventions to decrease the incidence of healthcare-associated *Clostridium difficile* infection. *Infection Control and Hospital Epidemiology, 30*(11), 1062–1069.

Abbett and colleagues tested prevention and treatment bundles to decrease the incidence of *Clostridium difficile* infection and the associated mortality at their tertiary-care, university-affiliated hospital. Over 1,047,849 patient-days, the rate of *C. difficile* infection dropped from 1.10 cases per 1,000 patient days to 0.66 cases per 1,000 patient days, a 40% reduction in incidence.

McDonald, L. C., Lessa, F., Sievert, D., Wise, M., Herrera, R., Gould, C., . . . Cardo, D. (2012). Vital Signs: Preventing *Clostridium difficile* infections. *Morbidity and Mortality Weekly Report, 61*(09), 157–162.

In this report, population-based data from the Emerging Infections Program are analyzed by location and prior healthcare exposures to better understand the contribution of nonhospital healthcare exposures to the overall burden of *C. difficile*. The report also explores the ability of programs to prevent *C. difficile* infection by implementing recommendations made by the Centers for Disease Control and Prevention. The results suggest that nearly all *C. difficile* infections are related to various healthcare settings where predisposing antimicrobials are prescribed and *C. difficile* transmission occurs. Results also show that an emphasis on infection control was successful at preventing hospital-onset infections.

Dubberke, E. R., Carling, P., Carrico, R., Donskey, C. Loo, V. G., McDonald, L. C., . . . Gerding, D. N. (2014). Strategies to prevent *Clostridium difficile* infections in acute care hospitals. *Infection Control and Hospital Epidemiology, 35*(6), 628–645.

In this compendium, the authors highlight some of the practical recommendations for acute care hospitals in their efforts to prevent *Clostridium difficile* infection. Using the most up-to-date evidence and presented in a concise format, strategies for *C. difficile* infection identification, prevention, and treatment are reviewed.

Hsu, J., Abad, C., Dinh, M., & Safdar, N. (2010). Prevention of endemic healthcare-associated *Clostridium difficile* infection: Reviewing the evidence. *The American Journal of Gastroenterology, 105*(11), 2327–2329.

In this systematic review of interventions to reduce healthcare-associated *Clostridium difficile* infection, the authors found that few randomized controlled trials exist for *C. difficile* infection prevention. The best evidence, however, suggests that antimicrobial stewardship, glove use, hand hygiene, and disposable thermometers should be routinely used for the prevention of *C. difficile* infection. The authors add that while potentially effective, environmental disinfection and probiotics require further investigation before their role in infection prevention can be determined.

The Future of Infection Prevention

I hate predictions, especially about the future.

—YOGI BERRA

The future of the struggle to prevent healthcare-associated infection (HAI), like its present, has two major ingredients—the adaptive and the technical. In this chapter we discuss both, though, as in the previous chapters, our emphasis is on the adaptive, behavioral change. That is not to slight the technical possibilities, a number of which could significantly reduce HAI as a serious problem. It's just that some of the adaptive possibilities could be put to work immediately, if only the healthcare community had the will to do so, whereas many of the technical items are years away from fruition.

The first development we would like to address is essentially adaptive, but it has a technical side as well. As previously discussed, we have conducted many interviews with hospital personnel, on the telephone and during site visits, to find out why some hospitals are more successful than others in combating catheter-associated urinary tract infection (CAUTI), ventilator-associated pneumonia (VAP), and central line-associated bloodstream infection (CLABSI). In that process, we have identified a number of common barriers to success, most of them related to the adaptive requirements of a quality improvement initiative, and we have also identified some common solutions. Ideally, hospitals having trouble should have the benefit of individual counseling, but that is unrealistic, given the hundreds of hospitals that might need assistance at any given time. So we have developed a CAUTI-specific "Guide to Patient Safety" (GPS) to help hospitals identify and cope with adaptive problems. The trouble-shooting system consists of two parts: a series of 14 yes/no, self-diagnostic questions about a hospital's CAUTI initiative, and feedback with suggested solutions tailored to that hospital's responses.

What makes the CAUTI GPS technical is that the list of questions and our responses can be accessed on the website www.catherout.org, a production primarily of the VA Ann Arbor Healthcare System and the University of Michigan Health System. We envision that the GPS will eventually be entirely web based, and the guidance will be automated. We also hope that the GPS will be expanded to include VAP, CLABSI, and other patient safety issues such as falls or *C. difficile*—and that it will aid hospitals about to embark on a quality initiative, not just those in the middle of one.

Meanwhile, you can check out the GPS in its current form, dealing with CAUTI, at www.catheterout.org, and in Box 10.1 you will find a copy of the GPS questionnaire. In some ways, the GPS also serves as a recap of much of the material presented in this book.

KEEPING PATIENTS OUT OF HOSPITALS

One reasonable response to the increase in infections acquired in hospitals, of course, is to keep chronically ill, infection-susceptible patients out of hospitals. The Centers for Medicare and Medicaid Services addressed that goal in 2012 when it began trimming payments to hospitals whose readmission rates for patients with a heart attack, congestive heart failure, or pneumonia were higher than predicted. Growing numbers of hospitals and insurers are arranging for many of these patients to be cared for in their own homes. Physicians and nurses visit patients daily and, when necessary, a variety of diagnostic and treatment options

Box 10.1 CAUTI PREVENTION GUIDE TO PATIENT SAFETY (ADAPTED FROM SAINT ET AL.[1])

1. Do you currently have a well-functioning team (or work group) focusing on CAUTI prevention?
   ☐ Yes ☐ No

2. Do you have a project manager with dedicated time to coordinate your CAUTI prevention activities?
   ☐ Yes ☐ No

3. Do you have an effective nurse champion for your CAUTI prevention activities?
   ☐ Yes ☐ No

4. Do bedside nurses assess, at least daily, whether their catheterized patients still need a urinary catheter?
   ☐ Yes ☐ No

5. Do bedside nurses take initiative to ensure the indwelling urinary catheter is removed when the catheter is no longer needed (e.g., by contacting the physician or removing the catheter per protocol)?
   ☐ Yes ☐ No

6. Do you have an effective physician champion for your CAUTI prevention activities?
   ☐ Yes ☐ No

7. Have physicians fully embraced CAUTI prevention activities?
   ☐ Yes ☐ No

8. Is senior leadership supportive of CAUTI prevention activities?
   ☐ Yes ☐ No

9. Do you currently collect CAUTI-related data (e.g., urinary catheter prevalence, urinary catheter appropriateness, and infection rates) in the unit(s) in which you are intervening?
   ☐ Yes ☐ No

(continued)

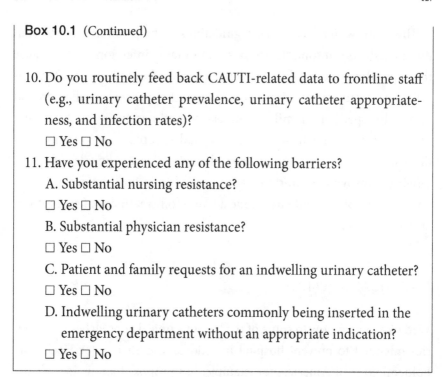

Box 10.1 (Continued)

10. Do you routinely feed back CAUTI-related data to frontline staff (e.g., urinary catheter prevalence, urinary catheter appropriateness, and infection rates)?
    ☐ Yes ☐ No
11. Have you experienced any of the following barriers?
    A. Substantial nursing resistance?
    ☐ Yes ☐ No
    B. Substantial physician resistance?
    ☐ Yes ☐ No
    C. Patient and family requests for an indwelling urinary catheter?
    ☐ Yes ☐ No
    D. Indwelling urinary catheters commonly being inserted in the emergency department without an appropriate indication?
    ☐ Yes ☐ No

are available in the home, from x-rays and echocardiograms to oxygen therapy and intravenous antibiotics. One study that compared the cost of treating similar patients at home and in a hospital reported that home care was 19% less expensive with equal or better outcomes.[2]

Another nonhospital site, the nursing home, presents a special challenge with regard to infection prevention, one that has attracted too little scientific attention in the past. Older patients typically have a variety of urogenital concerns, so urinary tract infection is common in these facilities—and so is catheterization. Urinary obstruction and impaired bladder emptying caused by stroke or diabetes may require the use of indwelling urinary catheters, part of the reason why a third of those who spend a year in a nursing home develop a urinary tract infection.[3] In addition, antimicrobials are frequently used automatically when infection is suspected through urinalysis, even though the patient may be asymptomatic and there is no medical reason to treat most patients who have asymptomatic bacteriuria with an antimicrobial.[4] Doing so only increases the probability that the patient will develop an antibiotic-resistant infection as well as increasing medical costs.

There are widely recognized guidelines to help nursing home staff distinguish asymptomatic from symptomatic infection, but because these usually require asking patients a series of questions about symptoms, communication difficulties make the process challenging at best. Also, patients' family members sometimes insist on treatment of asymptomatic bacteriuria with a broad-spectrum antimicrobial; as discussed in the previous chapter, that way lies *C. difficile* infection. Quality improvement initiatives are needed to reduce the use of Foleys and antimicrobials and encourage a hands-off treatment of asymptomatic bacteriuria.

TECHNICAL ADVANCES

We'd like to turn now to some of the latest technical approaches and theories intended to prevent hospital infections. The Society for Healthcare Epidemiology of America, for example, has proposed a new-look future for hospital clinicians' attire as a means to reduce the role of clothing in the spread of infection.[5] Its guidelines call for nonsurgical staff to be "bare below the elbows," wearing short sleeves and eschewing wristwatch, jewelry, and neckties during clinical practice as these items can become contaminated with antimicrobial-resistant bacteria. In hospitals that wished to maintain the wearing of the traditional, long-sleeved white coat, hooks would be provided upon which the coats would be hung before a clinician had direct contact with a patient.

One much-discussed approach is the use of devices that have a coating of silver and other antimicrobial materials, including urinary and central venous catheters and endotracheal tubes. The evidence for their effectiveness is mixed—strong for preventing CLABSI, uncertain for VAP, and weak for CAUTI. In 2009, we conducted a national survey of infection preventionists in more than 400 hospitals[6] and found what appeared to be only a limited correspondence between the evidence of effectiveness and the actual usage pattern of antimicrobial devices. Antimicrobial urinary catheters were reported in regular use in 45% of hospitals; antimicrobial central venous catheters in 33% of hospitals; and silver-coated endotracheal tubes in 5% of hospitals.

Why the widespread use of devices with only mixed scientific support? One possible answer was our survey's discovery that hospitals that regularly use an antimicrobial device to combat one HAI also tended to use such a device to combat another type of infection. The use of antimicrobial central venous catheters almost tripled the odds that a hospital would also be using antimicrobial *urinary* catheters.[7]

An additional reason for the popularity of the coated devices may be the simplicity of their application—switching uncoated for coated. And our investigations of quality improvement initiatives suggested yet a third possible explanation. Some hospitals gladly pay the extra cost of the devices, seeking to substitute a technical fix for the adaptive challenges of a quality initiative. The problem is that the devices by themselves cannot bring about the changed behaviors necessary to prevent most hospital infections.

Copper has powerful antimicrobial properties—copper-coated surfaces have been proven to cut the presence of bacteria by 99.9% in two hours. In one hospital study,[8] copper surfaces substantially reduced the contamination on frequently touched items such as door push plates and tap handles. Another study,[9] in an outpatient clinic, revealed a halo effect: Copper trays and arms fitted to a phlebotomy chair not only showed a 90% microbial reduction compared to noncopper trays and arms, but also reduced the contamination on their cloth-surfaced chairs by 70%. What has kept hospitals from embracing copper? Primarily, its high cost relative to other materials. And despite copper's proven antimicrobial power, clinical data have not shown a reduced risk in HAI—just because it kills bacteria on the surface, does not mean that it will lead to lower infections in humans. There is a third limiting factor: Because its antimicrobial effect takes a while, copper-coated surfaces are not so effective on toilet seats or other such surfaces where contamination takes place too frequently or too heavily.[8]

The increased focus on infection prevention has inspired a spurt of invention in the field of environmental disinfection, especially given the

growing scientific consensus that the hospital environment plays a significant role in the transmission of antimicrobial-resistant bacteria. The new
devices include robots that emit ultraviolet rays and various arrangements
that pump cleansing gases into a room. Tests of a Canadian system that
releases a vapor composed of ozone and hydrogen peroxide in a sealed
room[10] have achieved a 100% microbial kill rate in several hospital rooms
contaminated with methicillin-resistant *Staphylococcus aureus* (MRSA).
The vapor formula echoes nature: The human immune system generates
an ozone-hydrogen peroxide mix to combat germs.

A relatively simple technical device that could have an adaptive impact
in infection prevention is in the works at the University of Michigan.
It calls for all temporary devices inserted in a patient to carry a microchip, which would communicate with a series of three lights—green, yellow, and red—set above every hospital bed. The microchip would be set
according to the particular patient's requirements; for example, a situation
where the Foley should be withdrawn from the patient within 24 hours.
The green light would shine until the 24-hour period was drawing to a
close, when the yellow light would shine; finally, the red light would take
over. Each microchip would have its own frequency so that, if a patient
had two catheters (a Foley and a central venous catheter, for example),
there would be two sets of lights and no crossing of signals. The premise
behind the device is that physicians and nurses might bypass directions on
a patient's chart or a reminder on their pagers, but they would have a hard
time ignoring those lights shining in their eyes.

COMBATING DRUG-RESISTANT BACTERIA

Much of today's infection prevention effort on the technical side is inevitably
focused on drug-resistant bacteria like MRSA and carbapenem-resistant
Enterobacteriaceae (CRE) because infections caused by these bacteria are
becoming increasingly difficult to treat with currently available antibiotics. For example, researchers are developing new niche antibiotics that
specifically target patients with antibiotic-resistant infections. Supporters

are calling for the federal government to provide extra financial support and to create a limited approval pathway for these drugs, shortcutting the traditional large and long-term clinical trials.

Monoclonal antibodies are laboratory-produced antibodies designed to destroy disease cells without damaging healthy tissue. They have long since been used to treat cancer and rheumatoid arthritis and to prevent transplant rejection; they had global sales of more than $50 billion in 2012.[11] Now, scientists are exploring the use of these man-made antibodies to fight drug-resistant infections, including MRSA and CRE. Some monoclonal antibodies have successfully hindered the growth of S. aureus, encouraging the immune system to destroy the bacteria with phagocytes (cells that ingest foreign particles and debris). Molecules necessary to the survival of the drug-resistant bacteria are being attacked by other monoclonal antibodies, a strategy that makes it less likely that the bacteria will be able to mutate to withstand new antibiotics. One group of researchers has developed an antibody vaccine aimed at preventing MRSA from eroding bone around an orthopedic implant; the vaccine targets a protein necessary for bacterial growth.[12]

Other drugs are being tested that bypass the bacteria themselves, seeking to lessen the body's response to bacterial infection or deny the bacteria access to the body's resources. Healthy bacteria in the skin have been found to be the body's first-line of defense against MRSA. Therefore, some scientists are investigating whether oral doses of probiotics, live micro-organisms including some bacteria that may have health benefits, will reduce S. aureus nasal and gastrointestinal colonization. Probiotics are also being looked at as a treatment for CRE.

Scientists are testing faster and more accurate ways to diagnose infections, advances that may help clinicians better judge when and whether to use antibiotics. Instead of relying only on direct clinical symptoms, some researchers are measuring biomarkers released by the body in response to infection. High concentrations of serum procalcitonin, for example, may signal infection, including life-threatening urosepsis. In one study,[13] every member of a group of patients with a high procalcitonin level was shown to have severe bacterial urosepsis, a far more rapid diagnosis than by traditional means.

Researchers have suggested a new reason to cut back the use of antibiotics. Their studies have led them to suspect that the same antibiotics that have been so successful in increasing the growth of livestock and poultry may have the same effect on humans. Perhaps, they say, antibiotics may be partly responsible for the epidemic of obesity in the United States.[14]

New drug-delivery systems that obviate the need for catheters and ventilators may play a key role in the future prevention of infections. Nanomedicine, for example, may make it possible to release antibiotics precisely at an infection site deep within the body. Nanomachines have already proven capable of clamping interior arteries and tying sutures in animal studies.

PATIENTS AND PROVIDERS: A CHANGING RELATIONSHIP

Some of the most important and challenging aspects of healthcare's future, including the future of infection prevention, involve the relationship between patients and their healthcare providers. It has long been a relationship of unequals, with nurses and especially physicians holding the upper hand. That has been particularly evident in the hospital setting, where patients tend to be even more vulnerable and dependent. As diagnosis and treatment options have expanded with the new technology and patients have gained increased access to medical information, the relationship has begun to change. Patients are taking control of their own health in corporate wellness programs, learning from TV medical shows, and researching health issues on the Internet. In some health systems with electronic medical records, patients have electronic access to their own health records and can communicate directly with their physicians. Important health discussions are taking place around water coolers and in schools and community centers. At the same time, public agencies and medical organizations are calling for more of a partnership between doctor and patient—for patient empowerment.

To some extent, what we're seeing today is a confirmation of the theories of Geert Hofstede, a Dutch social psychologist. He studied the ways in which nations differ according to a group of values that include masculinity versus femininity and indulgence versus restraint. One of the values was the willingness of a country's less powerful citizens to accept the existing distribution of power, the status quo. On Hofstede's so-called Power Distance Index, Russia scored 93, indicating a high degree of acceptance, whereas Great Britain, Switzerland, Australia, the United States, and Canada had scores between 35 and 40. Citizens of the lower-ranking countries, Hofstede said, "strive to equalize the distribution of power."

American physicians who do infection prevention work in countries high on the Power Distance Index such as Japan soon become aware of the difference between their patients' attitudes toward medical authority and the attitudes of their U.S. patients. Studies show that in the United States today, both patients and healthcare providers favor greater patient and family participation in their own treatment. Both parties believe that increased patient participation can improve hospital safety and bring about better medical results in general. But studies also show that both parties tend to place limits on that participation.

It's one thing for physicians to explain the various treatment options to their patients, but few physicians are willing to have patients make the final treatment decision. We saw in earlier chapters how hospital patients and their families can complicate caregivers' efforts to have unnecessary Foleys removed, insisting that the convenience of the indwelling catheter is more important than the risk of infection it represents and the delay in surgical rehabilitation it can cause. Patients are not equipped by training or experience to take control over their medical treatment. In fact, research indicates that they have no burning desire to do so.

More and more patients do want to be informed about the various aspects of their diagnosis and treatment. Many of them are willing to become more active in monitoring both their own physical condition and the hospital care they receive. But they tend to back away from empowerment when it calls for them to decide among treatment options or to confront their providers. In some studies, patients were urged to ask caregivers about to have direct contact with them, "Did you wash your hands?" Most patients had trouble complying. One study[15] found that when a group of hospital patients was willing to confront caregivers, it paid dividends—a 50% increase in handwashing. In that case, all the participating patients were able to put the question to nurses, but just 35% asked it of doctors.

The patient empowerment movement is a relatively new phenomenon, and there is little scientific evidence about its effectiveness—but it does have substantial momentum. In the future, we suspect, hospital patients will become more aggressive in their own behalf, and physicians and nurses will become more comfortable with patients who ask a lot of questions and don't hesitate to express their opinions. We also expect that more clinical providers will move beyond a standardized approach, devoting extra time and effort to understanding and treating each patient as a singular individual with his or her own particular needs.

Encouragement to engage with patients arises not just from the patients themselves. A variety of public and private agencies and organizations have adopted that cause. The Choosing Wisely campaign is a relatively recent example, originally conceived by the National Physicians Alliance, taken up by the American Board of Internal Medicine (ABIM) Foundation, and joined by Consumer Reports. This is how the organization describes the campaign goal:

Choosing Wisely aims to promote conversations between physicians and patients by helping patients choose care that is:

- Supported by evidence
- Not duplicative of other tests or procedures already received
- Free from harm
- Truly necessary

The campaign has solicited from national organizations representing every major medical specialty a list of five common tests or procedures that "physicians and patients should question." We see it as no accident that in the adult Hospital Medicine category, the very first item reads, in part: "Don't place, or leave in place, urinary catheters for incontinence or convenience or monitoring of output for non-critically ill patients." The

Society of General Internal Medicine has added a list of its own to the Choosing Wisely initiative with five commonly ordered but not always necessary tests or procedures. The fifth item in the list may also strike a familiar note: "Don't place, or leave in place, peripherally inserted central catheters for patient or provider convenience." These lists are being widely distributed and promoted across the country, and Consumer Reports is creating patient-friendly materials to help patients prepare for their conversations with caregivers.

There is also a need to prep clinicians. In their interactions with patients, as in the other aspects of their lives, today's physicians and nurses are too often on autopilot, their minds preoccupied with thoughts of decisions to be made, calls to be returned, or an uncertain diagnosis. That kind of mental multitasking is a universal trait, of course, but in recent years it has been on the rise among hospital care providers, in part because of unrelenting and ever-increasing job pressures. One study[16] found that 46% of U.S. physicians reported at least one symptom of burnout. Clinicians are sometimes listening to patients with half an ear, thinking of one thing while doing another, reacting rather than responding.

THE POTENTIAL OF MINDFULNESS

To relieve the stress and get off autopilot, a growing number of healthcare providers are practicing mindfulness, the ability to be totally present and attentive in their lives and in their encounters with patients. The approach has its roots in Buddhist meditation, and its focus is on the processes of the mind. Its modern, secular incarnation, a blend of the teachings of yoga and Buddhism, was developed in part by Jon Kabat-Zinn, a molecular biologist by training, who is the founding executive director of the Center for Mindfulness in Medicine, Health Care, and Society at the University of Massachusetts Medical School. His mindful meditation classes are taught at medical centers around the world.

In those classes, clinicians learn how to achieve a beginner's mind, seeing everything, and every patient, as though for the first time, afresh. They learn how to observe themselves in the moment: Are they taking into account the whole context of the visit to a patient? Are they giving the patient a full chance to describe his or her symptoms and feelings? Are they fully attentive to the needs of the particular patient, undistracted by other thoughts and concerns and refusing to get stuck in the rut of their own expertise?

The few existing studies of the efficacy of mindfulness in a medical setting have reported generally positive results. One such paper[17] called for a group of physicians, nurse practitioners, and physician assistants to take a standardized written test gauging their level of mindfulness. They were then audio-recorded in encounters with patients, and the patients were later asked to rate the clinicians on the encounters. Those with high scores for mindfulness were more likely to have a patient-centered pattern of communication and a more positive emotional tone; they also received higher satisfaction ratings from their patients.

A major barrier to the widespread adoption of mindfulness by clinicians is time: Classes typically range from a week to a full day once a week for eight weeks. However, another study[18] of physicians who had taken an abbreviated mindfulness class—one weekend and two evening sessions—turned up similar results. The doctors were less anxious and depressed, and they remained so almost a year later.

Various aspects of mindfulness have been applied to improve patient safety and clinical practice. Present-moment awareness, for example, has been used in the primary care setting, and mindful control of cognitive biases has been suggested as a means to cut back diagnostic mistakes. We have developed a conceptual approach that we call mindful evidence-based practice. We believe that the mindful focus on clinicians' thinking processes may be helpful in implementing infection prevention initiatives, and we have designed a model (Figure 10.1) that illustrates that concept. In the model, mindful practice is shown as a cognitive process that moves from the clinician's individual values and experience through awareness of the patient's issue to careful consideration of the treatment options. The model also includes a clinical application: The mindful, experience-based cognitive process to determine whether an indwelling urinary catheter should be used.

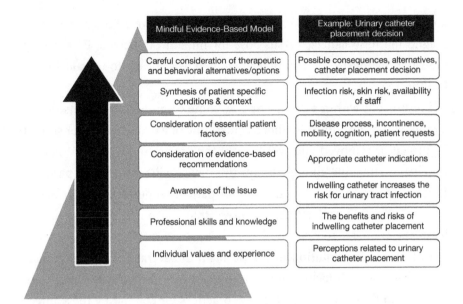

Figure 10.1
Mindful Evidence-Based Model (from Kiyoshi-Teo et al.[19])

In this chapter, we have had the audacity to offer some thoughts about what the field of infection prevention might look like in the decades to come. As the great management guru Peter Drucker once commented, "Trying to predict the future is like trying to drive down a country road at night with no lights on while looking out the back window." We recognize that we have only lightly touched on the multitude of technical advances that are in development. On the adaptive side, in particular, what we have written here about the future represents our hopes at least as much as our expectations.

One item we have neglected to mention that does not represent our hopes, but that seems to be an inevitable part of the future of medicine is IBM's Watson computer. IBM claims that the Watson can take in and analyze huge amounts of data better than humans, including physicians, and is thus just about ready to start making medical diagnoses. When confronted with a patient, the computer will be able to call up any and all of the relevant peer-reviewed medical knowledge of the past, as well as the latest research, all this to a degree no human doctor can match. This ability, one study found,[20] enabled Watson to achieve a 90% accuracy in diagnosing lung cancer, versus 50% for human physicians. By deriving the right diagnosis, the computer is touted as a means to drastically cut healthcare costs.

Presumably, within a decade or two, some combination of Watson and a robot will be deciding whether a central line or a urinary catheter should be placed or removed and will then fit the action to the word. What we find hard to imagine, though, is how this device will interact with patients. It doesn't seem to leave much room for patient empowerment, or for the human empathic and intuitive powers that machines have—so far, at least—been unable to muster.

In fact, the key solution to the problem of several hospital infections today lies less with technology than it does with the human dimension. We need to find a way to get the best practices for combating these infections put into clinical practice universally, and to do that we need a model to follow. In the previous chapters, we have presented such an adaptive model, using CAUTI as our main example. Because CAUTI impacts patients all through a healthcare system, from ICU to nursing home, and because it impacts a broad spectrum of hospital personnel, from nurses to microbiologists, the CAUTI model can be widely applied. And it can be used not just for preventing other infections like *C. difficile* but also for such other challenges as falls and pressure ulcers.

In closing, we would like to thank you for joining us on this journey. If what you have read has helped you to move forward in your struggle to conquer healthcare-associated infection, our mission will have been achieved.

SUGGESTIONS FOR FURTHER READING

Kiyoshi-Teo, H., Krein, S. L., & Saint, S. (2013). Applying mindful evidence-based practice at the bedside: Using catheter-associated urinary tract infection as a model. *Infection Control and Hospital Epidemiology, 34*(10), 1099–1101.
    In this article, the authors introduce a mindful, evidence-based practice model that illustrates how mindfulness might be used to incorporate evidence-based

practices into patient care at the individual clinician level. Using CAUTI prevention as an example, they illustrate how clinicians can be more mindful about appropriate catheter indications and timely catheter removal.

Borg, M. A. (2014). Cultural determinants of infection control behavior: Understanding drivers and implementing effective change. *Journal of Hospital Infection, 86*(3), 161–168.

In this article, the author focuses on three Hofstede constructs as necessary for improving infection prevention and control campaigns. In particular, he notes that many current infection prevention tools are strongly compatible with cultures that are low in uncertainty avoidance and power distance, and high in individualism and masculinity, a cultural combination that is largely restricted to Anglo-Saxon countries, where most of the recent improvements in HAI incidence have taken place.

Saint, S., Gaies, E., Harrod, M., Fowler, K. E., & Krein, S. L. (2014). Brief Report: Introducing a catheter-associated urinary tract infection prevention "Guide to Patient Safety" (GPS). *American Journal of Infection Control, 42*(5), 548–550.

Based on extensive qualitative evaluations, the authors developed a self-assessment tool called a CAUTI Guide to Patient Safety (or "CAUTI GPS"). In this article, they describe the rationale, features, and utility of such a quality improvement tool.

Salmon, P., & Hall, G. M. (2004). Patient empowerment or the emperor's new clothes. *Journal of the Royal Society of Medicine, 97*(2), 53–56.

In this article, Salmon and Hall explore the validity of "empowerment" as a concept by studying the experience of patients who have been empowered to take control and make choices. Based on these accounts from the patients' perspective, the authors suggest that patients do not generally embrace empowerment and that, in emphasizing research into how to empower patients at the expense of research into what patients feel like when they have been "empowered," medicine paradoxically continues the tradition of assuming that doctor knows best.

Spelberg, B., Bartlett, J. G., & Gilbert, D. N. (2013). The future of antibiotics and resistance. *New England Journal of Medicine, 368*(4), 299–302.

In this article, the authors propose future strategies to combat antimicrobial resistance. They suggest that long-term solutions require novel approaches based on a reconceptualization of the nature of resistance, disease, and prevention, and that additional societal investment in basic and applied research and policy activities is imperative.

REFERENCES

CHAPTER 1. A NEW STRATEGY TO COMBAT HOSPITAL INFECTIONS

1. Harbath, S., Sax, H., & Gastmeier, P. (2003). The preventable proportion of noso-comial infections: An overview of published reports. *Journal of Hospital Infection*, 54(4), 258–266.
2. Umscheid, C. A., Mitchell, M. D., Doshi, J. A., Agarwal, R., Williams, K., & Brennan, P. J. (2011). Estimating the proportion of healthcare-associated infections that are reasonably preventable and the related mortality and costs. *Infection Control and Hospital Epidemiology*, 2(2), 101–114.
3. Magill, S. S., Edwards, J. R., Bamberg, W., Beldavs, Z. G., Dumyati, G., Kainer, M. A., . . . Fridkin, S. K. (2014). Multistate point-prevalence survey of health care-associated infections. *New England Journal of Medicine*, 370(13), 1198–1208.
4. Scott, R. D. II. (2009). The direct medical costs of healthcare-associated infections in U.S. hospitals and the benefits of prevention. (Publication number CS200891-A). Atlanta, GA: Centers for Disease Control and Prevention. Retrieved from http://www.cdc.gov/hai/pdfs/hai/scott_costpaper.pdf.
5. Stone, P. W., Pogorzelska-Maziarz, M., Herzig, C. T. A., Weiner, L. M., Furuya, E. Y., Dick, A., & Larson, E. (2014). State of infection prevention in US hospitals enrolled in the National Health and Safety Network. *American Journal of Infection Control*, 42(2), 94–99.
6. Michigan Health & Hospital Association Patient Safety and Quality. (2012). *Annual Report 2012*. Retrieved from http://www.mhakeystonecenter.org/documents/2012psqreport.pdf

CHAPTER 2. COMMITTING TO AN INFECTION PREVENTION INITIATIVE

1. Saint, S., Meddings, J. A., Calfee, D. P., Kowalski, C. P., & Krein, S. L. (2009). Catheter-associated urinary tract infection and the Medicare rules changes. *Annals of Internal Medicine*, 150, 877–885.
2. Lee, G. M., Hartmann, C. W., Graham, D., Kassler, W., Dutta-Linn, M., Krein, S., . . . Jha, A. (2012). Perceived impact of the Medicare policy to adjust payment for health care-associated infections. *American Journal of Infection Control*, 40(4), 314–319.

3. Saint, S., Olmsted, R. N., Fakih, M. G., Kowalski, C. P., Watson, S. R., Sales, A. E., & Krein, S. L. (2009). Translating health care-associated urinary tract infection prevention research into practice via the bladder bundle. *Joint Commission Journal on Quality and Patient Safety, 35*(9), 449–455.

4. Hartocollis, A. (May 29, 2013). With money at risk, hospitals push staff to wash hands. *New York Times*, p. A18.

CHAPTER 3. TYPES OF INTERVENTIONS

1. Erasmus, V., Daha, T. J., Brug, H., Richardus, J. H., Behrendt, M. D., Vos, M. C., & van Beeck, E. F. (2010). Systematic review of studies on compliance with hand hygiene guidelines in hospital care. *Infection Control and Hospital Epidemiology, 31*(3), 283–294.

2. Saint, S., Lipsky, B. A., Baker, P. D., McDonald, L. L., & Ossenkop, K. (1999). Urinary catheters: What type do men and their nurses prefer? *Journal of the American Geriatric Society, 47*(12), 1453–1457.

3. Cornia, P. B., Amory, J. K., Fraser, S., Saint, S., & Lipsky, B. A. (2003). Computer-based order entry decreases duration of indwelling urinary catheterization in hospitalized patients. *American Journal of Medicine, 114*(5), 404–407.

4. Saint, S., Kaufman, S. R., Thompson, M., Rogers, M. A., & Chenoweth, C. E. (2005). A reminder reduces urinary catheterization in hospitalized patients. *Joint Commission Journal on Quality and Patient Safety, 31*(8), 455–462.

5. Gould, C. V., Umscheid, C. A., Agarwal, R. K., Kuntz, G., Pegues, D. A. & Healthcare Infection Control Practices Advisory Committee. (2010). Guideline for prevention of catheter-associated urinary tract infections 2009. *Infection Control and Hospital Epidemiology, 31*(4), 319–326.

6. Meddings, J., Rogers, M. A., Krein, S. L., Fakih, M. G., Olmsted, R. N., & Saint, S. (2014). Reducing unnecessary urinary catheter use and other strategies to prevent catheter-associated urinary tract infection: An integrative review. *BMJ Quality and Safety, 23*(4), 277–289.

7. Srinivasan, A., Wise, M., Bell, M., Cardo, D., Edwards, J., Fridkin, S., . . . Pollock, D. (2011). Vital signs: Central line-associated bloodstream infections—United States, 2001, 2008, and 2009. *Morbidity and Mortality Weekly Report, 60*(08), 243–248.

8. Pronovost, P., Needham, D., Berenholtz, S., Sinopoli, D., Chu, H., Cosgrove, S., . . . Goeschel, C. (2006). An intervention to decrease catheter-related bloodstream infections in the ICU. *New England Journal of Medicine, 355*(26), 2725–2732.

9. Render, M. L., Hasselbeck, R., Freyberg, R. W., Hofer, T. P., Sales, A. E., Almenoff, P. L., & Group, V. I. C. A. (2011). Reduction of central line infections in Veterans Administration intensive care units: An observational cohort using a central infrastructure to support learning and improvement. *BMJ Quality and Safety, 20*(8), 725–732.

10. Gawande, A. (2009). *The checklist manifesto: How to get things right.* New York, NY: Metropolitan Books.

11. Kress, J. P., Pohlman, A. S., O'Connor, M. F., & Hall, J. B. (2000). Daily interruption of sedative infusions in critically ill patients undergoing mechanical ventilation. *New England Journal of Medicine, 342*(20), 1471–1477.

12. Smith, G. C., & Pell, J. P. (2003). Parachute use to prevent death and major trauma related to gravitational challenge: Systematic review of randomised controlled trials. *BMJ (Clinical Research), 327*(7429), 1459–1461.

CHAPTER 4. BUILDING THE TEAM

1. Health care personnel flu vaccination: Internet panel survey, United States, November 2012. Retrieved from http://www.cdc.gov/flu/fluvaxview/hcp-ips-nov2012.htm

2. Fakih, M. G., Krein, S. L., Edson, B., Watson, S., R., Battles, J., B., & Saint, S. (in press). Engaging healthcare workers to prevent catheter-associated urinary tract infection and avert patient harm. *American Journal of Infection Control.*

3. Farley, J. E., Doughman, D., Jeeva, R., Jeffries, P., & Stanley, J. M. (2012). Department of Health and Human Services releases new immersive simulation experience to improve infection control knowledge and practices among health care workers and students. *American Journal of Infection Control, 40*(3), 258–259.

4. Krein, S. L., Kowalski, C. P., Harrod, M., Forman, J., & Saint, S. (2013). Barriers to reducing urinary catheter use: A qualitative assessment of a statewide initiative. *JAMA Internal Medicine, 173*(10), 881–886.

CHAPTER 5. THE IMPORTANCE OF LEADERSHIP AND FOLLOWERSHIP

1. American College of Healthcare Executives. (2013). Top issues confronting hospitals: 2013. Chicago, IL. Retrieved from http://www.ache.org/pubs/research/ceoissues.cfm

2. Collins, J. (2001). *Good to great: Why some companies make the leap. . . and others don't.* New York, NY: HarperCollins.

3. Northouse, P. (2013). *Leadership: Theory and practice* (6th ed.). Thousand Oaks, CA: SAGE.

4. Association of American Medical Colleges. (2011). Addressing the physician shortage under reform. Washington, DC: Mann. Retrieved from https://www.aamc.org/newsroom/reporter/april11/184178/addressing_the_physician_shortage_under_reform.html

5. Saint, S., Kowalski, C. P., Banaszak-Holl, J., Forman, J., Damschroder, L., & Krein, S. L. (2010). The importance of leadership in preventing healthcare-associated infection: Results of a multisite qualitative study. *Infection Control and Hospital Epidemiology, 31*(9), 901–907.

6. Mayer, J. D., & Salovey, P. (1997). What is emotional intelligence? In P. Salovey & D. J. Sluyter (Eds.), *Emotional development and emotional intelligence* (pp. 3–31). New York, NY. Basic Books.

7. Kelley, R. E. (1992). *The power of followership.* New York, NY: Doubleday Currency.

8. Van de Waal, E., Borgeaud, C., Whiten, A. (2013). Potent social learning and conformity shape a wild primate's foraging decisions. *Science, 340*, 483–485.

9. Rogers, E. M. (2003). *Diffusion of innovations* (5th ed.). New York, NY: Free Press.

CHAPTER 6. COMMON PROBLEMS, REALISTIC SOLUTIONS

1. Pascale, R., Sternin, J., & Sternin, M. (2010). *The power of positive deviance: How unlikely innovators solve the world's toughest problems.* Boston, MA: Harvard Business Review Press.

2. Reinertsen, J. L., Gosfield, A. G., Rupp, W., & Whittington, J. W. (2007). *Engaging physicians in a shared quality agenda.* IHI Innovation Series white paper. Cambridge, MA: Institute for Healthcare Improvement. (Available on www.IHI.org)

3. Saint, S., Kowalski, C. P., Banaszak-Holl, J., Forman, J., Damschroder, L., & Krein, S. L. (2009). How active resisters and organizational constipators affect health care-acquired infection prevention efforts. *Joint Commission Journal on Quality and Patient Safety, 35*(5), 239–246.

4. Saint, S., Wiese, J., Amory, J. K., Bernstein, M. L., Patel, U. D., Zemencuk, J. K., ... Hofer, T. P. (2000). Are physicians aware of which of their patients have indwelling urinary catheters? *The American Journal of Medicine, 109*(6), 476–480.

5. Harrod, M., Kowalski, C. P., Saint, S., Forman, J., & Krein, S. L. (2013). Variations in risk perceptions: A qualitative study of why unnecessary urinary catheter use continues to be problematic. *BMC Health Services Research, 13,* 151. doi: 10.1186/1472-6963-13-151

6. Grant, A. M., & Hofmann, D. A. (2011). It's not all about me: Motivating hand hygiene among health care professionals by focusing on patients. *Psychological Science, 22*(12), 1494–1499.

CHAPTER 7. TOWARD SUSTAINABILITY

1. Miller, B. L., Krein, S. L., Fowler, K. E., Belanger, K., Zawol, D., Lyons, A., ... Saint, S. (2013). A multimodal intervention to reduce urinary catheter use and associated infection at a Veterans Affairs Medical Center. *Infection Control and Hospital Epidemiology, 34*(6), 631–633.

2. Lieber, S. R., Mantengoli, E., Saint, S., Fowler, K. E., Fumagalli, C., Bartolozzi, D., ... Bartoloni, A. (2014). The effect of leadership on hand hygiene: Assessing hand hygiene adherence prior to patient contact in 2 infectious disease units in Tuscany. *Infection Control and Hospital Epidemiology, 35*(3), 313–316.

3. Pronovost, P. J., Goeschel, C. A., Colantuoni, E., Watson, S., Lubomski, L. H., Berenholtz, S. M., ... Needham, D. (2010). Sustaining reductions in catheter-related bloodstream infections in Michigan intensive care units: Observational study. *BMJ Clinical Research, 340,* c309.

CHAPTER 8. THE COLLABORATIVE APPROACH TO PREVENTING INFECTION

1. ØVretveit, J., Bate, P., Cleary, P., Cretin, S., Gustafson, D., McInnes, K., ... Wilson, T. (2002). Quality collaboratives: Lessons from research. *Quality and Safety in Health Care, 11*(4), 345–351.

2. Nembhard, I. M. (2009). Learning and improving in quality improvement collaboratives: Which collaborative features do participants value most? *Health Services Research, 44*(Part 1), 359–378.

3. Schouten, L. M., Hulscher, M. E., van Everdingen, J. J., Huijsman, R., Grol, R. P. (2008). Evidence for the impact of quality improvement collaboratives: Systematic review. *British Medical Journal, 336*(7659), 1491–1494.

CHAPTER 9. TAKING ON *C. DIFFICILE*

1. Johnson, S., Gerding, D. N., Olson, M. M., Weiler, M. D., Hughes, R. A., Clabots, C. R., & Peterson, L. R. (1990). Prospective, controlled study of vinyl glove use to interrupt *Clostridium difficile* nosocomial transmission. *American Journal of Medicine, 88*(2), 137–140.
2. Grady, D. (March 20, 2012). Gut infections are growing more lethal. *New York Times*, p. D1.
3. Mayo Clinic. (2013). Diseases and conditions: C. *difficile* infection. Retrieved from http://www.mayoclinic.org/diseases-conditions/c-difficile/basics/definition/con-20029664
4. Eyre, D. W., Cule, M. L., Wilson, D. J., Griffiths, D., Vaughan, A., O'Connor, L., . . . Walker, A. S. (2013). Diverse sources of C. *difficile* infection identified on whole-genome sequencing. *New England Journal of Medicine, 369*(13), 1195–1205.
5. Dubberke, E. R., Gerding, D. N., Classen, D., Arias, K. M., Podgorny, K., Anderson, D. J., . . . Yokoe, D. S. (2008). Strategies to prevent *Clostridium difficile* infections in acute care hospitals. *Infection Control and Hospital Epidemiology, Supplement 1*, S81–S92.
6. Rotjanapan, P., Dosa, D., & Thomas, K. S. (2011). Potentially inappropriate treatment of urinary tract infections in two Rhode Island nursing homes. *Archives of Internal Medicine, 171*(5), 438–443.
7. Fridkin, S., Baggs, J., Fagan, R., Magill, S., Pollack, L. A., Malpied, P., . . . Srinivasan, A. (2014). Vital Signs: Improving antibiotic use among hospitalized patients. *Morbidity and Mortality Weekly Report, 63*(9), 194–200.
8. Flanders, S. A., & Saint, S. (2014). Why does antimicrobial overuse in hospitalized patients persist? *JAMA Internal Medicine, 174*(5), 661–662.
9. Spellberg, B. (2014). Antibiotic judo: Working gently with prescriber psychology to overcome inappropriate use. *JAMA Internal Medicine, 174*(3), 432–433.
10. Rousseau, J-J. (1762). *The social contract*. (Book 1, Section 7). London: Penguin.
11. Flanders, S. A., & Saint, S. (2012). Enhancing the safety of hospitalized patients: Who is minding the antimicrobials? Comment on "Overtreatment of Enterococcal Bacteriuria." *Archives of Internal Medicine, 172*(1), 38–40.
12. Abbett, S. K., Yokoe, D. S., Lipsitz, S. R., Badar, A. M., Berry, W. R., Tamplin, E. M., & Gawande, A. A. (2009). Proposed checklist of hospital interventions to decrease the incidence of healthcare-associated *Clostridium difficile* infection. *Infection Control and Hospital Epidemiology, 30*(11), 1062–1069.
13. Van Nood, E., Vrieze, A., Nieuwdorp, M., Fuentes, S., Zoetendal, E. G., de Vos, W. M., . . . Keller, J. J. (2013). Duodenal infusion of donor feces for recurrent *Clostridium difficile*. *New England Journal of Medicine, 368*(5), 407–415.

CHAPTER 10. THE FUTURE OF INFECTION PREVENTION

1. Saint, S., Gaies, E., Harrod, M., Fowler, K. E., & Krein, S. L. (2014). Brief Report: Introducing a catheter-associated urinary tract infection prevention "Guide to patient safety" (GPS). *American Journal of Infection Control, 42*(5), 548–550.

2. McCain, J. (2012). Hospital at home saves 19% in real-world study. *Managed Cared, 21*(11), 22–26.

3. Span, P. (April 7, 2011). A common infection, commonly overtreated. *New York Times*. Retrieved from http://newoldage.blogs.nytimes.com/2011/04/07/in-nursing-homes-a-common-infection-is-commonly-overtreated/?_php=true&_type=blogs&_r=0

4. Flanders, S. A., & Saint, S. (2012). Enhancing the safety of hospitalized patients: Who is minding the antimicrobials? Comment on "Overtreatment of Enterococcal Bacteriuria." *Archives of Internal Medicine, 172*(1), 38–40.

5. Bearman, G., Bryant, K., Leekha, S., Mayer, J., Munoz-Price, S., Murthy, R., . . . White, J. (2014). Healthcare personnel attire in non-operating-room settings. *Infection Control and Hospital Epidemiology, 35*(2), 107–121.

6. Krein, S. L., Kowalski, C. P., Hofer, T. P., & Saint, S. (2012). Preventing hospital-acquired infections: A national survey of practices reported by U.S. hospitals in 2005 and 2009. *Journal of General Internal Medicine, 27*(7), 773–779.

7. Saint, S., Greene, M. T., Damschroder, L., & Krein, S. L. (2013). Is the use of anti-microbial devices to prevent infection correlated across different healthcare-associated infections? Results from a national survey. *Infection Control and Hospital Epidemiology, 34*(8), 847–849.

8. Noyce, J. O., Michels, H., & Keevil, C. W. (2006). Potential use of copper surfaces to reduce survival of epidemic MRSA in the healthcare environment. *Journal of Hospital Infection, 63*(3), 289–297.

9. Rai, S., Hirsch, B. E., Attaway, H. H., Nadan, R., Fairey, S., Hardy, J., . . . Schmidt, M. G. (2012). Evaluation of the antimicrobial properties of copper surfaces in an outpatient infectious disease practice. *Infection Control and Hospital Epidemiology, 33*(2), 200–201.

10. Zoutman, D., Shannon, M., & Mandel, A. (2011). Effectiveness of a novel ozone-based system for the rapid high-level disinfection of health care spaces and surfaces. *American Journal of Infection Control, 39*(10), 873–879.

11. TransWorldNews. (November 30, 2013). Global monoclonal antibody market: $50 billion industry in 2012. Retrieved from http://www.transworldnews.com/1483738/a70079/global-monoclonal-antibody-market-50-billion-industry-in-2012

12. Varrone, J. J., Li, D., Daiss, J. L., & Schwarz, E. M. (2011). Anti-glucosaminidase monoclonal antibodies as a passive immunization for methicillin-resistant staphylococcus aureus (MRSA) orthopaedic infections. *Bonekey Osteovision, 8*, 187–194.

13. Mitsuma, S. F., Mansour, M. K., Dekker, J. P., Kim, J., Rahman, M. Z., Tweed-Kent, A., & Schuetz, P. (2013). Promising new assays and technologies for the diagnosis and management of infectious diseases. *Clinical Infectious Diseases, 56*(7), 996–1002.

14. Kennedy, P. (March 9, 2014). The fat drug. *New York Times*, p. SR1.

15. McGuckin, M., Waterman, R., Storr, I. J., Bowler, I. C., Ashby, M., Topley, K., & Porten, L. (2001). Evaluation of a patient-empowering hand hygiene programme in the UK. *Journal of Hospital Infection, 48*(3), 222–227.

16. Shanafelt, T. D., Boone, S., Tan, L., Dyrbye, L. N., Sotile, W., Satele, D., . . . Oreskovich, M. R. (2012). Burnout and satisfaction with work-life balance among U.S. physicians relative to the general U.S. population. *JAMA Internal Medicine, 172*(18), 1377–1385.

17. Beach, M. C., Roter, D., Korthuis, P. T., Epstein, R. M., Sharp, V., Ratanawongsa, N., . . . Saha, S. (2013). A multicenter study of physician mindfulness and health care quality. *Annals of Family Medicine, 11*(5), 421–428.

18. Fortney, L., Luchterhand, C., Zakletskaia, L., Zgierska, A., & Rakel, D. (2013). Abbreviated mindfulness intervention for job satisfaction, quality of life, and compassion in primary care clinicians: A pilot study. *Annals of Family Medicine, 11*(5), 412–420.

19. Kiyoshi-Teo, H., Krein, S. L., & Saint, S. (2013). Applying mindful evidence-based practice at the bedside: Using catheter-associated urinary tract infection as a model. *Infection Control and Hospital Epidemiology, 34*(10),1099–1101.

20. Steadman, I. (February 11, 2013). IBM's Watson is better at diagnosing cancer than human doctors. *Wired*. Retrieved from http://www.wired.co.uk/news/archive/2013-02/11/ibm-watson-medical-doctor/viewall

INDEX

Page numbers followed by *b, f,* or *t* indicate boxes, figures, or tables, respectively.

ABCDE recommendations, 16, 17*b*
ABIM Foundation. *See* American Board of Internal Medicine Foundation
accountability, 79
active resistance, 77–84, 88*b*
alienation, 62
American Board of Internal Medicine (ABIM) Foundation, 134
American College of Healthcare Executives, 53
ancient medicine, 20–21
Ann Arbor Healthcare System: CAUTI Cost Calculator, 12*b*
antimicrobial devices, 128–129
antimicrobial restrictions, 113–114, 115*b*–116*b*
antimicrobials, 82
antimicrobial stewardship, 114
antiseptics, 30*b*, 30
APIC. *See* Association for Professionals in Infection Control and Epidemiology
Aristotle, 91
Association for Professionals in Infection Control and Epidemiology (APIC), 23
Association of American Medical Colleges, 56
Association of Practitioners in Infection Control, 23

bacteria, drug-resistant, 6, 10, 130–132
balloon catheters, indwelling, 20–21
barriers to change, 86–89, 88*b*–89*b*
behavior, leadership, 59–62
Bennis, Warren, 57
Berra, Yogi, 124
Berwick, Donald, 67
bilevel positive airway pressure (BiPAP), 33
Bismarck, Otto von, 28
bladder bundles. *See also* bundle instructions
    for preventing CAUTI, 25–26, 34
    for preventing CAUTI in ICU, 50–51
Bleichröder, Fritz, 28
bloodstream infections. *See* central line-associated bloodstream infection (CLABSI)
British Medical Journal, 33
bundle instructions
    "people bundle," 37–38
    postoperative order sets, 50
    for preventing *C. difficile* infection, 113–114
    for preventing CAUTI, 25–26, 34, 50–51
    for preventing CLABSI, 34
    for preventing VAP, 32
bundle theory, 101–102

campaign messages, 46

carbapenem-resistant *Enterobacteriaceae* (CRE), 130–131

catheter-associated urinary tract infection (CAUTI), 3–5, 24–28
  CAUTI Cost Calculator, 12*b*
  claims data, 13
  costs of, 12*b*
  "Guide to Patient Safety" (GPS), 125, 126*b*–127*b*
  prevention bladder bundles, 25–26, 34, 50–51
  prevention guide to patient safety, 125, 126*b*–127*b*
  prevention in the ED, 49–50
  prevention in the ICU, 50–51
  prevention model, 6
  recommendations for preventing, 16, 17*f*
  treatment of, 20–21

catheter patrol, 94

catheters
  Foley, 5, 24–26, 50
  history of, 20–21
  indwelling, 5, 20–21, 71–72, 73*t*

CAUTI. *See* catheter-associated urinary tract infection

CAUTI Cost Calculator, 12*b*

CDI (*Clostridium difficile* infection), 111–123

CDI (*Clostridium difficile* infection) checklist, 118, 119*t*–121*t*

Centers for Disease Control and Prevention (CDC), 23, 112–113

Centers for Medicare and Medicaid Services (CMS)
  Hospital Compare website, 10–11
  hospital reimbursements, 4, 12–13, 24, 125–127
  incentives, 12–15

central line-associated bloodstream infection (CLABSI), 28–31
  claims data, 13
  prevention bundle, 34
  prevention practices, 3

Central Line Infection Prevention Checklist, 30*b*, 30

central lines (central venous catheters), 5, 129

CEOs (chief executive officers), 15–18, 53–55

checklists. *See also* bundle instructions
  C. difficile infection (CDI) checklist, 118, 119*t*–121*t*
  Central Line Infection Prevention Checklist, 30*b*, 30
  daily, 50
  "Guide to Patient Safety" (GPS), 125, 126*b*–127*b*
  postoperative order sets, 50

chief executive officers (CEOs), 15–18, 53–55

chiefs of staff, 59

Choosing Wisely initiative, 134–135

CLABSI. *See* central line-associated bloodstream infection

clinicians, 128

Clostridium difficile, 112–113

Clostridium difficile infection (CDI), 111–123

Clostridium difficile infection (CDI) checklist, 118, 119*t*–121*t*

clothing, 128

CMS. *See* Centers for Medicare and Medicaid Services

collaboration, 100–110

collegiality, 14

Collins, Jim, 54

communication, 46
  patient-friendly materials, 135
  patient-physician conversations, 134–135

Comprehensive Hospital Infections Project, 23

conformists, 62

Consortium for Research on Emotional Intelligence in Organizations, 62

constipators, organizational, 84–86

Consumer Reports, 134–135

copper-coated surfaces, 129

costs
  of CAUTIs, 12*b*
  of HAIs, 2–3
CRE (carbapenem-resistant *Enterobacteri
  aceae*), 130–131
culture, hospital, 14–15

daily catheter patrol, 94
daily checklists, 50
data collection, 42, 42*f*, 44*t*
Deming, W. Edwards, 101
Diffusion of Innovations (Rogers), 65
discipline, 109
disease: germ theory of, 21–22
disinfection, environmental, 130
doctors. *See* physicians
Drucker, Peter, 1, 5–6, 137
drug-delivery systems, 132
drug-resistant bacteria, 6, 10, 130–132

early planning, 92–93
ED (emergency departments), 49–50
educational posters, 46
egalitarianism, 14
emergency department (ED), 49–50
emotional intelligence, 61
emotional quotient (EQ), 61–62
empowerment, 134
Enterobacteriaceae, carbapenem-resistant
  (CRE), 130–131
environmental disinfection, 130
evaluations, monthly, 94
evidence-based medicine, mindful, 136,
  137*f*
executive concerns, 53
executive decisions, 15–18
executive sponsors, 42–43
exemplary followers, 63

feedback, 101
financial challenges, 53
financial incentives, 2–3, 12*b*, 13
Foley, Frederic Eugene Basil, 20–21
Foley catheters, 5, 24–25
  alternatives to, 26, 84

"discontinue Foley," 50
  insertion of, 26
  "presence/rationale for Foley," 50
Foley Police or Foley Patrol, 48
followers, 53–69
follow-up meetings, 47–48
Franklin, Benjamin, 20–21
Franklin, John, 20–21
future directions, 124–139

Gandhi, Mohandas K., 70
germ theory, 21–22
Good to Great and the Social Sectors
  (Collins), 54
government mandates, 53
GPS. *See* "Guide to Patient Safety"
group norms, 64–65
groups, 64–68
guidance, 71–72, 74*t*
"Guide to Patient Safety" (GPS), 125,
  126*b*–127*b*

HAIs. *See* healthcare-associated infections
hand hygiene
  bladder bundle, 25–26
  Central Line Infection Prevention
    Checklist, 30*b*, 30
  maintaining progress in, 96–97
Harvard Business Review, 62
healthcare-associated infections (HAIs)
  costs of, 2–3
  interventions against *C. difficile,* 118,
    119*t*–121*t*
  prevalence of, vii, 2–3
  prevention of, 2, 124–139
healthcare providers, 132–135. *See also*
  nurses; physicians
healthcare reform, 53
Hippocrates, 111
history
  of catheters, 20–21
  of infection control, 22–24
Hofstede, Geert, 132–133
Homer, 101
hospital attire, 128

hospital clinicians, 128
Hospital Compare website (CMS), 10–11
hospital culture, 14–15
hospital infections, 21–22
    germ theory of disease, 21–22
    new strategy against, 1–8
hospitalists, 41
hospital leaders, 58–59, 66–67
hospitals
    CMS reimbursements to (Medicare
        payments), 4, 12–13, 24, 125–127
    model, 25–26, 102–103
Huxley, Thomas Henry, 20
hygiene, hand
    bladder bundle, 25–26
    Central Line Infection Prevention
        Checklist, 30b, 30
    maintaining progress in, 96–97

IBM, 137–138
ICUs. *See* intensive care units
IHI. *See* Institute for Healthcare
    Improvement
implementation teams, 37–52
incentives
    CMS, 12–15
    financial, 2–3, 12b, 13
    hospital, 10–12
indwelling catheters (Foley), 5, 20–21
    removal of, 71–72, 73t, 75t
infection prevention
    collaborative approach to, 100–110
    future directions, 124–139
    history of, 22–24
    types of interventions, 20–36
infection prevention initiatives, 9–19
infection preventionists, 41–42
infections
    C. difficile, 111–123
    catheter-associated urinary tract
        infection (CAUTI), 3–5, 24–28
    central line-associated bloodstream
        infections (CLABSI), 3, 28–31
    healthcare-associated, vii, 2–3
    hospital, 1–8

ventilator-associated pneumonia
    (VAP), 3, 31–33
initiatives
    infection prevention initiatives, 9–19
    Keystone ICU Initiative, 29, 97
    nursing initiatives, 71–72, 74t
Institute for Healthcare Improvement
    (IHI), 24, 28
Institute of Medicine (IOM), 24
intensive care unit (ICU) directors, 56
intensive care units (ICUs), 3
    CLABSI rates, 29
    Keystone ICU Initiative, 29, 97
    preventing CAUTI in, 50–51
interventions
    barriers and possible solutions, 71–72,
        73t–75t
    against *C. difficile* infections, 118,
        119t–121t
    infection prevention initiatives, 9–19
    Keystone ICU Initiative, 29, 97
    nursing initiatives, 71–72, 74t
    types of, 20–36
IOM. *See* Institute of Medicine
Ishikawa, Kaoru, 101

JAMA Internal Medicine, 115b
Joint Commission on Accreditation of
    Hospitals, 23–24

Kabat-Zinn, Jon, 135
Kelley, Robert E., 62
Keystone ICU Initiative, 29, 97
Kocher, Gerhard, 4
Krein, Sarah, 4

Lao Tzu, 57
leadership, 53–69
    barriers and possible solutions, 71–72,
        74t, 79
    "hire hard, manage easy" school, 59
    key traits, 57, 57b
    "management by walking around"
        approach, 58
    transactional, 54–55, 55b

transformational, 54–55, 55*b*
Lister, Joseph, 22
Locke, John, 115*b*

management by walking around, 58
managers, 57. *See also* project managers
Mayer, John, 61
MDROs (multi-drug resistant
    organisms), 10
Mead, Margaret, 37
Medicare payments, 4, 12–13, 24,
    125–127
meetings, first, 45–47
methicillin-resistant *Staphylococcus
    aureus* (MRSA), 6, 10, 130–131
Michigan Health and Hospital
    Association, 4, 29, 97
microchips, 130
mindfulness, 135–138, 137*f*
monitoring, 42, 44*t*
Montgomery, Bernard, 53
monthly evaluations, 94
MRSA (methicillin-resistant *Staphylococc
    us aureus*), 6, 10, 130–131
multi-drug resistant organisms
    (MDROs), 10

nanomachines, 132
nanomedicine, 132
Nanus, Burt, 57
Napoleon, Bonaparte, 57
National Fascist Party, 102
National Healthcare Safety Network
    (NHSN), 13, 23
National Nosocomial Infections
    Surveillance System (NNIS), 23
National Physicians Alliance, 134
National Surveillance System for
    Healthcare Workers, 23
new treatments, 122
NHSN. *See* National Healthcare Safety
    Network
Nightingale, Florence, 9
NNIS. *See* National Nosocomial
    Infections Surveillance System

noninvasive positive-pressure ventilation
    (NPPV), 32–33
nonprofits, 54–57
Northouse, Peter G., 57
NPPV (noninvasive positive-pressure
    ventilation), 32–33
nurse champions, 38–39, 44*t*, 83–84
nurses, 4, 71–72, 73*t*, 74*t*, 82
    resistant, 81, 83–84
    scheduling, 71–72, 74*t*
nurse supervisors, 46
nursing initiatives, 71–72, 74*t*
"100,000 Lives" campaign, 24, 28

organizational constipators, 84–86, 88*b*

passivists, 63
Pasteur, Louis, 22
patient empowerment movement, 134
patient-friendly materials, 135
patient-provider relationships, 132–135
patient safety, 53
    "Guide to Patient Safety" (GPS), 125,
        126*b*–127*b*
"people bundle," 37–38
physician champions, 40–43, 44*t*
physician-patient relationships, 132–135
physicians, 71–72, 73*t*, 74*t*, 77–80
    older, 79
    resistant, 71–72, 77, 75*t*, 79–81
physician shortage, 56
planning, early, 92–93
pneumonia, ventilator-associated
    (VAP), 3, 31–33
positive airway pressure, bilevel
    (BiPAP), 33
positive-pressure ventilation, noninvasive
    (NPPV), 32–33
posters, educational, 46
postoperative order sets, 50
power, 133
Power Distance Index, 133
pragmatists, 63
prevention guide to patient safety, 125,
    126*b*–127*b*

prevention initiatives, 9–19
prevention of infection, 2
  CAUTI model, 6
  Central Line Infection Prevention
    Checklist, 30b, 30
  collaborative approach to, 100–110
  in the ED, 49–50
  future directions, 124–139
  in the ICU, 50–51
  initiatives for, 9–19
  protective measures against *C. difficile*,
    116–122
  recommendations for preventing
    CAUTI, 16, 17f
  suggestions for further reading, 7–8
  types of interventions, 20–36
prevention teams, 114–116
  duties of, 93–96
  implementation teams, 37–52
problem solving, 70–90
program sustainability, 91–99
project managers
  first team meeting, 46–47
  roles and responsibilities, 42–43, 44t
project teams
  duties of, 93–96
  implementation teams, 37–52
  prevention teams, 114–116
promotion, 54
protective measures, 116–122
public relations, 46

quality improvement, 53
  active resisters to, 77–84
  barriers and possible solutions, 71–72,
    73t–75t
  challenges, 71–72
  financial incentives for, 13
quality improvement collaboratives
  18-month project, 104–106
  advantages of, 108–109
  cookie-cutter experience of,
    106–108
  Japanese beginnings, 101–102
quality improvement initiatives, 13, 43

randomized controlled trials, 33–34
recruitment, 38–39
reminders, 80
reminder systems, 26–27, 27f
reporting, 42, 44t
resistance to change
    active, 77–84, 88b
    solutions for, 71–72, 77, 75t, 79
resistant bacteria, 6, 10, 130–132
resistant nurses, 81, 83–84
resistant physicians, 81
resources: suggestions for further read-
    ing, 7–8, 18–19, 34–36, 51–52,
    68–69, 89–90, 97–99, 109–110, 123,
    138–139
Rogers, Everett M., 64–66
Rousseau, Jean-Jacques, 115b

safety concerns, 53
safety guide, 125, 126b–127b
Saint, Sanjay, 4
Salovey, Peter, 61
scheduling, 71–72, 74t
SCIP (Surgical Care Improvement
    Project), 95
Semmelweis, Ignaz, 21
SENIC Project (Study on the Effectiveness
    of Nosocomial Infection
    Control), 23–24
sepsis, 6
The Social Contract (Rousseau), 115b
Society for Healthcare Epidemiology of
    America, 128
Society of General Internal Medicine, 135
staff, 11, 72, 75
    challenging styles, 86–89, 88b–89b
    chiefs of staff, 59
staff attire, 128
staff recruitment, 38–43
staff turnover, 59
standard operating procedures, 26
Staphylococcus, 6
Staphylococcus aureus, methicillin-resistant
    (MRSA), 6, 10, 130–131
stewardship, antimicrobial, 114

stop orders, 28
strengththroughunity.org
    website, 101–102
Study on the Effectiveness of Nosocomial
    Infection Control (SENIC
    Project), 23–24
Surgical Care Improvement Project
    (SCIP), 95
sustainability, 91–99

team building, 37–52
team duties, 93–96
team managers, 42–43, 44*t*
team meetings
    first, 45–47
    follow-up, 47–48
team members, 42–43, 44*t*
team operations, 43–48
teams
    implementation teams, 37–52
    prevention teams, 114–116
    project teams, 93–96
technical advances, 128–130
time management, 136
timeservers, 86–89, 89*b*

"To Err Is Human" (IOM), 24
transactional leadership, 54–55, 55*b*
transformational leadership, 54–55, 55*b*
turnover, 59

University of Michigan, 12*b*, 130
urinary catheter data collection sheets, 42,
    42*f*
urinary catheter reminders, 26–27, 27*f*
urinary catheters
    antimicrobial, 129
    indwelling, 5, 71–72, 73*t*
urinary management policy, 26
urinary tract infection. *See*
    catheter-associated urinary tract
    infection (CAUTI)

ventilation, noninvasive positive-pressure
    (NPPV), 32–33
ventilator-associated pneumonia
    (VAP), 3, 31–33
ventilators, 5
Veterans Administration (VA), 12*b*
Veterans Health Administration
    (VHA), 27, 29